EBURY PRESS

THE ASTHMA CURE

Tarika Ahuja is an international wellness coach with over fourteen years of experience in natural medicine and macrobiotics. She has worked in New York, Austin, Santa Monica, Becket, Mangaluru, Bengaluru, Ludhiana, Chennai, New Delhi, Gurugram and Rishikesh, as well as Belgium and Spain.

Ahuja is dedicated to making an integrated and efficient system of wellness available for all, especially children. Her work with women and children is particularly notable. Her own healing journey inspired her to come up with Sacred Swan, an organization that supports women and children working towards happiness and creative fulfilment.

The Asthma Cure is her second book, after *Beautiful Children*.

THE ASTHMA CURE

A holistic macrobiotic and Ayurvedic guide to stronger lungs, resilient immunity, gut health and healthy weight

TARIKA AHUJA

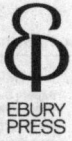

EBURY
PRESS

An imprint of Penguin Random House

EBURY PRESS

USA | Canada | UK | Ireland | Australia
New Zealand | India | South Africa | China | Singapore

Ebury Press is an imprint of the Penguin Random House group of companies
whose addresses can be found at global.penguinrandomhouse.com

Published by Penguin Random House India Pvt. Ltd
4th Floor, Capital Tower 1, MG Road,
Gurugram 122 002, Haryana, India

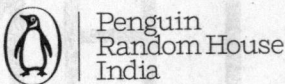

First published in Ebury Press by Penguin Random House India 2018

ISBN 9780143444312

Typeset in Adobe Caslon Pro by Manipal Digital Systems, Manipal

Printed at Manipal Technologies Limited, India

www.penguin.co.in

*To my nephews, nieces and the future
generation of wellness warriors
who will hopefully spread the message
and advice in this book*

Contents

Contents

Foreword

Asthma is related to one's diet and environment. Most dietary issues revolve around the production of excess mucus and inflammation. The major contributing factors of asthma and other lung diseases are dairy products and sugar, including substitutes like high-fructose syrups. These foods tend to cause inflammation and swelling in the bronchial tubes, besides leading to the production and secretion of mucus. This makes normal breathing difficult and often leads to a chronic condition. With this condition as the platform, a reverse reaction—a muscle spasm—occurs. That is an asthma attack.

Air pollutants only worsen this condition. When the bronchial tubes swell up and are coated with sticky mucus, the respiratory system cannot discharge particulates efficiently. They stick to the inner bronchial tubes and cause further inflammation. Many children in India and China, where air pollution is accelerating, are prone to this condition.

Modern medicine currently has no cure for asthma. Bronchial dilators are very strong muscle relaxing agents that offer only temporary relief. Even though medication and dilators help relax the strong contractions of the bronchial tubes during an attack, if used regularly they can weaken and inflame the lungs even more, thereby leaving an individual prone to even more attacks. Therefore, we can say that dilators are a temporary solution that is harmful in the long run.

What we need is a long-term solution with dietary change as the foundation. The change needs to involve a move away from animal fats and sugars and towards a plant-based diet. It also involves consuming foods that work towards dissolving excess mucus in the body and reversing the weakness and inflammation in the lungs.

Traditional energy medicine—such as yoga, macrobiotics, Ayurveda, naturopathy, Unani—had a very clear understanding about specific mucus-dissolving vegetables, which have now been lost. Besides consuming a healthy diet, which may be plant-based or plant-exclusive depending on an individual's values and choices, there are certain roots, seeds, medicinal concoctions and condiments that help pull out the mucus from the lungs and reverse inflammation. Taking care of your diet and purifying your blood helps minimize the damage inflicted by air pollution and other common triggers.

If we apply the information in this book with diligent consistency, the results will be self-evident. I have known Tarika for over thirteen years now and she has always been a deep thinker. She has an exceptional sensitivity, intelligence and dedication towards holistic health. Her caring nature and genuine concern for individual and planetary health is creditable. Not everyone has the ability to see things the way she does. Her message through this book can help solve the growing problem of lung and respiratory diseases, and create a generation of strong and healthy individuals.

Edward Esko
author, macrobiotic educator and founder of
the International Macrobiotic Institute

Introduction

For all of you suffering from asthma or any other respiratory disease, I wish to share genuine and practical information that would help improve or heal your condition. Today, people have lost the ancient knowledge and deep intuitive sagacity about life, health and nature. I must add that neglecting this ancient wisdom and nature-based life principles has only caused us harm.

Change Is a Constant Factor in Our Lives

Nothing is static. We change constantly. Every action, thought and choice we make; every person, school, organization or philosophy we encounter, leaves an impression on us. It may be active influence or subtle, a positive impression or negative. Similarly, the things we eat also affect us on many levels: physical, mental, emotional and spiritual. We may or may not be aware of all the consequences of our daily actions, which may not manifest instantaneously but will surely do so over a period of time. Whichever way, change is inevitable and constant and directly linked to our daily lives, environment and choices.

Over a period of time, our daily choices have a cumulative effect. We must make healthy choices. What we choose affects our body, mind, health, digestive sensitivity, blood quality, physical strength, immune function, work, relationships, mood and much more.

What Is Health?

Usually people refer to health as the result mentioned in a medical report or pain (or its absence) in the body. Yes, these are obvious and active signs of health. But these are not the only indications. We are simply unaware of the other signs. Our facial features, skin texture, blemishes, marks, pimples, hair quality, eyes and lips all speak volumes about what is happening inside of us. All of these change on a daily, weekly, monthly and yearly basis. You could say that our ability to heal and change our negative state depends on the choices we make. For example, a person's cheeks are indicative of the health of his or her lungs. If the lungs are weak, the cheeks may appear discoloured, suffer loss of elasticity, become enlarged, drooping, or become prone to pimples, blemishes or freckles. Similarly, the lips represent the digestive system. The upper lip corresponds to the stomach and the lower lip represents the lower digestive system, i.e., the intestines. Reddish or swollen lips may be a sign of inflammation while dark lips may represent blood stagnation.

Over months and years of a well-guided holistic wellness practice, this can change for the better.

Energy Medicine Is More than Simple Nutrition

Our choices should be informed and must come from a good understanding of our body type and energy balance instead of just nutritional information. An understanding of the relationship between the energy provided by the food we eat and our body type is a more holistic approach to making healthy choices. Sometimes we think that we are doing everything we should for our health, but often it isn't organized, methodical or consistent enough to have a lasting effect. It makes more sense to study food as energy medicine rather than as nutrition to see a visible and lasting impact. It also makes more sense to think of food as more than just nutrients or calories. Besides scientific nutrition, everything we eat has its own unique energy, certain inherent qualities, nature and behaviour. How it acts in nature is how it will act within us. For example, stalks of grain resemble the human spine. Hence eating wholegrains helps to heal and develop our brain and spinal functions. Besides wholegrains containing nutrients and fibre, they have other qualities that are passed on to us when we consume them. This is referred to as energy medicine which is a combination of nutrition and other factors.

Initially, we may need to work with professional health counsellors and follow authentic guidelines based on dependable systems of healing. But what are these systems of healing? They are systems based on a profoundly comprehensive system of energy such as Ayurveda, macrobiotics, yoga, posture alignment and techniques to de-stress the mind, etc. A holistic counsellor or educator does not limit healing to food and lifestyle changes but looks deeply into other aspects of one's life, including stress, posture and spinal health, emotions, relationships, possible environmental toxins and passion for one's work.

These systems of healing are nature-based and, like everything else in nature, they work gradually. They don't offer quick fix solutions. Yes, food gives us energy, but it can also be used in an organized and methodical way to be medicinal. When it comes to food, it is the repeated intake of healing food that makes it medicinal. The energy contained in food is gentle and subtle. It requires one to keep up intake of healing foods on a daily basis for months so that it can have a visible impact on the organ concerned. Having one healthy meal or a few meals, or including a few health supplements, can be beneficial but not medicinal. Having a few good meals a week has little impact as opposed to a consistent and methodical diet that leads to health and healing. Using food as a medicine requires a certain level of understanding of the relationship between food and its curative qualities.

Genetic Predisposition vs Current State of Health

Every human being is born with a certain constitution and body type. Our constitution is largely defined by our genetic structure and what our mother consumed during pregnancy. You could also say that our genetic propensities and body type is a predisposition that we are born with. Though this has an impact on our life, generally speaking, it is our daily choices and environment that have a greater impact on us.

Essentially, besides our genetic structure or body type, we also have a current state of condition. Our current condition changes with time and is different from our constitution. Our constitution has a lasting general impact throughout our life whereas our condition changes every day based on our daily choices. Our blood plasma changes every ten days, our white blood cells change every two to three weeks and our red blood cells change every 120 days. Most of our organs change every two years and our entire body goes through a substantial change every seven to ten years.

Is Asthma Incurable?

Asthma is a combination of both our current condition and genetic predisposition. Some diseases are influenced by time-dependent lifestyle choices. Genetics play a smaller role in such cases. However, for people suffering from asthma, there may be a significant genetic factor involved. If that is the case, it may contribute to slow healing, requiring more effort and a multidimensional approach. This often leads to the impression that asthma is incurable thus leaving people to rely on suppressive rather than curative interventions. Modern medicines suppress symptoms while traditional systems such as macrobiotics and Ayurveda aim to cure the disease.

Asthma is a curable disease. This is the primary reason why I chose to write this book; and I hope to work as an asthma revolutionary through workshops and awareness campaigns in order to break the myth that it is incurable.

An adult with asthma or a family with an asthmatic child often become so overwhelmed by the degree or frequency of attacks or discomfort that they have little energy left to dive deeper into the root cause. And understandably so because after a while, they run out of patience and motivation to make any extra effort. They are content as long as they can manage it. Life becomes an unending struggle for them, all because of the belief that the disease is incurable.

This book helps you explore the deeper causes of asthma and provides a simple step-by-step approach to what can help cure it. The book shares knowledge about medicinal roots and food combinations that dry out excessive mucus in the body while reducing inflammation and strengthening the lungs.

The Two Evils of Asthma

The underlying cause of asthma is excessive mucus production and high-degree inflammation. An individual with asthma cannot afford to let the mucus production and inflammation increase. They have to pick the right foods to control inflammation and excessive mucus production.

For asthma and respiratory tract-related ailments, it is important to cleanse the lungs and melt down the hard mucus buildup that causes blockages by not consuming foods that can trigger mucus production in the first place. To heal asthma, the lungs need to regain their strength and suppleness. Hence consuming a combination of the right foods and practising postures that help the lungs regain elasticity is important. To heal respiratory diseases, we need to strengthen the immune function and fight inflammation at every level every day.

What to Eat and What to Avoid

For an individual with asthma or any other respiratory disease such as chronic cough and allergies, bronchitis, emphysema, etc., dietary guidelines are not just about what to eat, but also about what to avoid. Thus merely eating the right kinds of foods is not enough. Many people eat foods and herbs that strengthen the lungs but do not remove those that increase the double evils of mucus production and inflammation. Hence they feel that all their efforts of using natural methods, herbs and supplements are slow and not as effective. This book talks extensively about the exact foods that can increase or decrease mucus production and inflammation depending on the severity and body type.

Improving Posture and Core Strength

All our organs are connected and nourish each other in a cyclical way. A poor posture leads to compression of organs and impedes circulation. An upper-body hunch that reduces blood circulation to the lungs and heart will affect the rest of the body too. Similarly, a weaker lower back which reduces circulation to the adrenals, kidneys and the gut affects the endocrine system and immune function. Improving posture, strengthening the abdominal core and working through the hip and leg joints is essential for the whole body. It's only when the core and lower-body joints are strong that the lungs can have a strong foundation which allows them to open up and breathe better. The book therefore also dwells on the importance of maintaining the correct posture as an essential part of the process to contain and heal lung diseases.

Stress and Asthma

According to traditional and ancient medicine philosophies, the emotions connected to the lungs are depression and stress. With weaker lungs, one is more easily pulled down by these emotions. Hence the importance of a healthy and emotionally supportive environment should be considered important.

A stressful environment affects everyone. A person with weak lungs or stomach is more sensitive to stress. These two systems—the ability to breathe and the ability to digest—are of prime importance as they transmute anything we take in into usable energy. With these two systems not functioning well, we live just one-tenth of our life's potential. Stress management and maintaining a happy environment is critical.

The Purpose of This Book: Dispelling Misinformation

I have been fortunate to come across some profound and rooted healing modalities in the world. Many of these support the healing process and can take you to the next best stage of health. Some healing systems are more powerful than others but have missing links in the sense that often the foundational information is either missing or isn't unified or complete. I personally feel that these systems are pure of intention, and perhaps temporarily effective, but simply not accurate. For a sensitive disease like asthma, we cannot afford inaccuracy as it leads to a loss of faith in the solution owing to ineffective results.

When you are privileged to study and understand the basis of reversing a disease, it compels you to share the information. Our future generations deserve to know better. I have completed the Macrobiotic Leadership Programme from Kushi Institute (which closed down in December 2016) and other health and healing programmes at the Natural Epicurean Academy of Culinary Arts, besides participating in certified advanced macrobiotic counselling programmes with renowned macrobiotic counsellor Verne Varona as well as one-on-one sessions with other teachers. I have also studied other healing and natural wellness medicinal programmes such as intuitive anatomy, reiki, Stott Pilates and yoga.

My intensive studies and practical experience have helped me understand healing from a deeper perspective. Of course, certain individuals may take longer than others to heal but that should not stop our efforts from moving in the right direction. This book is about creating support for all those suffering from asthma and other lung-related diseases. In fact, the basic guidelines in this book will help improve immunity and lung function of any individual, regardless of whether or not they suffer from asthma. Given the pollution in our times, all of us need to take care of our lungs and immunity.

The air in our cities is a lot more toxic than it used to be. Chronic exposure to high-degree pollution is a major reason behind the decline in proper functioning of the lungs and the respiratory system, and the increase in lung-related diseases. Our body assimilates much lesser oxygen from the air today than it did 100 years ago. In today's world taking better care of our lungs has become imperative.

All of us must seek to study and develop a deeper understanding of ourselves and our disease states. Based on the deep-rooted principles of macrobiotics, Ayurveda and yoga, this book aims to serve as a practical guidebook to help dispel misinformation and support your understanding of your health in a systematic way.

Macrobiotics and Asthma

1

What Is Macrobiotics?

'Macro' means large and 'biotic' means life. Macrobiotics is the practice of a large (great) and long life. It is often referred to as the practice of longevity. It's an ancient healing system—a lot like Ayurveda—that sees the body as a systematic web of energy rather than just a physical unit.

What makes this enormously sophisticated and complex human system function properly or poorly? There is a network of energy channels underlying the physical and visible systems. These channels follow a direction, some upwards and some downwards, some to the left and some to the right. If energy moves through the body in a stable and systematic way—in the original direction of these channels—then a person will experience health and balance. If for some reason there is an obstruction in any of these channels and the energy does not move in the way it is supposed to-but moves through the body in an unstable or chaotic way, then pain and disease conditions surface.

Macrobiotics is the practice of creating balance, keeping in mind the five elements of nature—wood or tree, fire, soil or earth, metal and water—and our connection to them. It is also about the balance between the contractive (masculine) and expansive (feminine) energies which every individual balances uniquely.

Often, certain cultures honour the feminine and denounce the masculine. There is a lot of ambiguity regarding these energies. Some people view the words 'masculine' and 'feminine' in a very emotional way. Both of them are relevant and necessary. Each individual has a unique combination of these. You can say that it is the balance between activity and rest. Both activity and rest are important in any individual's life and need to be balanced. If we are too active, it may lead to exhaustion and burnouts. On the contrary, if we rest too much, we may become sluggish, which will affect circulation. These opposite energies of expansion and contraction, also called yin and yang, are like dilation and constriction. We cannot afford to have our capillaries or blood vessels extremely constricted or extremely dilated. Health is in moderation, not in the extremes.

The way I see it is that we need to avoid both extremes. Extreme contraction or masculine energy may lead to rigidity, hardness and constriction in the body systems. In the event of a heart attack or asthma attack, the constriction is a result of extreme masculine energy. Healthy masculine energies are associated with strength and vitality. Healthy feminine energies are connected to flow, flexibility and relaxation, while extreme feminine energies are linked to weakness and fragility. For example, a weak nervous system, lungs or muscles are a sign of extreme feminine energies in the body. This shows that any extreme is bad and that balance is achieved by avoiding them. Therefore, the spiritual and cultural belief that endless expansion is good is faulty. Yes, we need to expand any contraction enough for it to be relaxed and flexible. But beyond a certain point, expansion becomes structureless and leads to weakness, disintegration and fragility.

While asthma as a chronic disease is normally associated with weak lungs or a chronic expansive (yin) condition of the lungs, an asthma attack is an extreme masculine (yang) condition of the bronchial tubes. Removing the extremes will definitely help improve one's condition. Generally, removing or reducing foods from the extreme categories listed in the table on the next page will help heal asthma and other lung-related diseases. Consuming more foods from the central column in a systematic and consistent way will help strengthen the lungs. You can say that macrobiotics is an intelligent, relevant and systematic approach to health and healing. In fact, apart from essential health and healing, it automatically leads a person towards a life of *Sattva*, which means a state of purity, wisdom and natural goodness.

Table 1(a)

Contraction (Yang)		Balance		Expansion (Yin)
Extreme Masculine	**Healthy Masculine**	**Balanced**	**Healthy Feminine**	**Extreme Feminine**
Rigidity	Strength	Health	Flexibility	Weakness
Hardness	Vitality	Flow	Relaxation	Disintegration of energy and health
Constriction				Fragility
Asthma attack				Chronically weak and inflamed lungs in asthma as a chronic disease

Table 1 (b)

Extreme Yang (Contraction)	Healthy Yang	Balance between the opposite energies	Healthy Yin	Extreme Yin (Expansion)
Examples of foods that cause contractions	**Examples of foods that give strength**	**Examples of foods that balance**	**Examples of foods that relax**	**Examples of foods that weaken the system**
Meat	Hearty soups and stews	Whole grains	Blanched/ steamed salad	White sugar
Poultry (chicken and eggs)	Sea vegetables	Beans and lentils	Raw salads	Refined foods

Excessive salt	Spirulina	Sweet vegetables	Sprouts	Soft dairy such as ice cream, butter, cream cheese
Excessively hard baked foods such as crackers, cookies, nachos	Root vegetables like kudzu, burdock and ginger	Root vegetables	Microgreens	Alcohol
Hard cheeses	White meat fish[1] (optional)	Ground vegetables	Fruits	Fruit juices (unseasonal combinations)
		Leafy green vegetables	Fruit juices (balanced and seasonal combinations)	Chemicals, preservatives in commercial foods
		Home-made fermented foods (with salt)	Raw honey (in moderation)	Drugs and other stimulants
			Organic ghee (in moderation)	Coffee

How I Came Across Macrobiotics . . .

In 2004, I secured admission and a partial scholarship at one of the best art schools in the US—SMFA (School of the Museum

---

[1] Quality of fish must be evaluated while choosing it.

of Fine Arts) in Boston. When I was visiting home during the winter break, my family insisted that I start exploring a project to work on rather than going to art school for four years. After giving this some thought, I decided to consider the idea of opening a vegetarian restaurant and a contemporary craft store in Goa. Somehow, I was always more inclined towards a plant-based diet. I was also quality-conscious and didn't want to work towards random goals. I wanted to study and understand the benefits of a balanced vegetarian diet. Back then, I hadn't even heard of macrobiotics. As a young girl, I was always conscious and sensitive, and also concerned with the quality of information I promoted, which is why I decided to gain in-depth knowledge about balanced vegetarian foods. Looking back, I thank my lucky stars for my innate ability to look deeper than just superficial nutritional information, even at such a young age!

One morning, at 4 a.m. during my winter break, I searched the Internet for vegetarian cooking schools (I typed the words 'vegetarian schools + USA' into the search bar. After all, I had a ticket back to the US after the winter break). I came across only three schools back then. Of these, two were *Macrobiotic*. What is macrobiotics? I wondered. It sounded like an unusual term. After further research, it seemed to be an interesting far-eastern philosophy. It was exotic and confusing at the same time. I signed up for two of the schools. One was in Austin, Texas, and the other one was in Becket, a small town in western Massachusetts.

I studied at these two schools under deeply intuitive teachers who had over thirty to forty years of experience in healing and reversing lifestyle and chronic diseases. They inspired me to bring all their wisdom and practical knowledge back to India. I was thrilled. To my surprise, I found out later that I was the first Indian to have studied at the Kushi Institute in Becket.

Studying for a year in an authentic macrobiotic environment helped me distinguish between what macrobiotics is and what it is not. The Internet had some careless and confusing information. At the school, we were taught by eight to ten teachers. Each teacher presented us with several case studies that helped us understand the subject better. The curriculum wasn't just centred around bookish knowledge. In fact, our teachers told us that macrobiotic teachings are 'non-credo', which means that one shouldn't give them credit till they experience the results. This made sense because reading a few articles on the Internet, though inspiring, can be misleading. Proper guidance through experts is a necessity to understand and apply this information well. All my teachers emphasized the importance of deep understanding and gave us good guidelines for daily practice so that we could see the results for ourselves. This is the intention of this book too—to impart practical guidelines. When practised long enough, they will give you your own understanding and results, leading to a certain level of conviction.

After studying under such inspiring teachers, I came back to India. Within a month, I met an old American lady named Mona Schwartz. She had been living and practicing macrobiotics in Dehradun. I was lucky to have been able to spend extensive quality time with her. She had a dynamic, warm and witty personality and had been trying to teach macrobiotics in India for many years. We kept in touch and worked towards common goals. A year or two later, I went back to my school in the US and studied with some teachers there. Not only did I have the good fortune to go to great schools, but I also studied with accomplished teachers. This gave me a unique in-depth understanding of macrobiotics. I

was indeed fortunate to have the gift of first-hand experience
with teachers across the globe.

Healthy Diet vs Healing Diet

The guidelines for a healthy diet are different from those for
a healing diet. Unfortunately, to a person not familiar with
these ideas eating healthy sounds like a lot like instructions
and restrictions. This is a flawed opinion. In fact, following
practical macrobiotic guidelines helps create more freedom:
freedom from a weak body, deficiencies and health or weight
imbalances. It leaves you with more energy to pursue your
dreams and goals. A healthy diet includes a wide range of
foods, cooking styles, flavours and cuisines. This is because
macrobiotics is not about flavours and cuisines alone. It is a
set of universally balanced energy-based principles which may
be applied to any country, cuisine or taste palate.

Variety Is an Essential Part of a Healthy Diet

It is not good for a person who eats the healthiest of foods to
repeat the same thing every day. For example, a healthy diet
consists of more grains than one. Some people have only rice,
or only wheat (as in chapatti), or both. This isn't enough. For
a healthy variety, it is good to include a minimum of three
to six grains—this is the minimum not the maximum. You
can choose from brown rice, black rice, red rice, white rice
(for occasional use), cracked wheat, wheat flour (for bread or
chapatti), cracked barley, whole barley or pearl barley, foxtail
millet, finger millet (ragi), barnyard millet, black millet (bajra),
buckwheat (for occasional use), corn, etc. Some of these are
recommended for daily cooking, while others are for weekly

or occasional use. Some may be boiled, some stir-fried, some as a salad, mashed, or made into patties and croquettes. There is nothing boring about wholegrains.

Healthy vegetables should be used more often in a variety of forms such as soup, salad, stir-fried, as traditional and delicious subzi or even raw. Each cooking method brings out a different nutritional value. One wouldn't get enough nutrition by having only soups and salads or having only subzis or overcooked veggies. We need to put different cooking and preparation methods to use. Different nutrients become available from the same food when they are cooked differently. It is also advisable to eat not only dals but also beans. Some households rotate between a few dals, but it is the variety that brings vitality. If a person or child is not fond of beans, one can make bean burgers or patties or even soups. Having beans is essential as dals alone do not provide enough nutrition and nourishment.

No Particular Herb or Cuisine Is Supreme or Favoured

It's not true that any one cuisine is better than other cuisines. For example, Thai food is not better than Italian or Japanese or Indian cuisine. You may cook using cumin (jeera), coriander, garam masala, sambar masala, coconut, lemongrass, rosemary or basil. Make coriander–mint chutney or idli podi or a tahini–lemon dressing or coconut–basil dip. You may have lemon or ginger or chilli pickle, as long as they are made at home or without toxic ingredients. Variety is always welcome, provided it is healthy. The key lies in the balance between the proportions and combinations used each day. To understand this better, you can go through the daily, weekly and occasional food list on pages 48 and 49.

A healing diet is very different from a healthy diet and may come with more restrictions. For example, if you are recovering from cancer or a liver disease or thyroid—or anything where the body needs specific foods as per one's body type and condition—then the diet may be restrictive for as long as eight to twelve months or as suggested by a macrobiotic or Ayurvedic counsellor. This is a temporary plan to heal a disease that must not be followed for a lifetime. Limited desserts, less spice and less oil may be recommended for some people. But these suggestions are temporary and not a clue as to what a healthy person should eat. Some people hear the suggestions offered to a cancer patient and think that macrobiotics is too limiting. It must be remembered that a healing diet is not a reflection of what a healthy diet is.

Macrobiotics Is More a Practice and Less a Philosophy

Macrobiotics is not just a philosophy like I thought it was. It is a practice. The philosophy is there to inspire action and have a larger understanding so that we can make better long-term choices and decisions. Coming across macrobiotics and studying its principles was like a blessing for me. These universal principles, if followed daily, can guide us for as long as we live.

An Artist Should Eat Different from a Banker or Athlete

As human beings, for whatever we wish to achieve—be it recovering from a disease, strengthening our immune function, being our best weight as per our genetic structure, or having the right intensity and energy to be an athlete, artist or leader—we need to adopt an action plan that matches our priorities and life goals. This is where macrobiotics is totally different from diets and nutrition plans. It isn't a set list of dos and don'ts. It is an understanding about the nature of different kind of foods and how they could possibly act and react in the human system. It is an understanding of the different body types, diseases and lifestyles, and matching guidelines to achieve results.

Macrobiotics Is Not a Diet

The term macrobiotics is not the name of a diet. As authors and educators, we often use the term 'diet' as an easy explanation when there is a lack of time to explain. In the true sense, macrobiotics is an intelligent application of a set of universal principles that can be applied to many things, including diet.

One man's medicine may be another man's poison. There is and should be a different approach for different people, with some basic guidelines in place. These common guidelines are the backbone of balance. However, variations apply as per a person's health, age, sex, local climate conditions and lifestyle. Hence, a diet to heal liver cancer is often different from someone trying to address asthma, hypertension or diabetes. One needs to invest a little time to study the subject and practise it in a way that works best for one's goals and body type. This may take six months for some and two years for some others. People looking for quick results in just a week or month seldom benefit from macrobiotics.

Macrobiotics also emphasizes on the opposites and how to balance them. For example, the balance between activity and rest, dry and wet, hot and cold, etc.

Macrobiotics helps us develop a profound understanding of the five elements of nature and how they affect our health,

mind, body, emotions, personality, facial features and all of
our energy. Every organ system corresponds to a particular
element, emotion and strength or weakness. Macrobiotics
also seeks to balance the opposite energies of contraction/
gathering and expansion/dispersion. It is an in-depth
understanding of the complex interplay of the five elements
and their corresponding action within us.

Nature isn't just beautiful scenery to admire. Our bodies,
minds, emotions and our connection to one another are
all affected by nature and its functioning. Nature isn't just
a concept of healing either, but is also our primary living
energy. Some people are aware of this direct and absolute
connection to the five elements and use this information to
maximize their health and potential. Many may think that
nature is beautiful and intuitively realize that it has a calming
effect on us. But they still may not be aware of the vast
potential of working closely with the five elements on a daily
basis. This is the depth, power and accuracy of macrobiotic
principles. Energy-based health isn't just about nutrients,
calories and diet plans. That isn't what macrobiotics is about.
Macrobiotics is not a partial system. It is a holistic system
that encompasses many aspects of our lives.

How Do Organs Affect Emotional Health?

As mentioned above, different organ systems are associated
with different elements. Similarly, different foods are
connected with different elements. For example, the element
'wood' is associated with the function of the liver and gall
bladder. It is connected to foods like barley, leafy greens and
spring-time foods (like leeks, scallions, celery, dandelion root).
Light, natural and sour flavours such as lemons and Granny

Smith apples also nourish the liver and gall bladder. Lightly cooked green vegetables and salads are also very nourishing. When these organs function well, a person is more likely to be patient, assertive and passionate. When these organs are clogged up, an individual may experience irritability, tension and outbursts. The liver and gall bladder are most harmed by excess animal protein, poor-quality or excessive animal fats or trans-fats and spicy food. They are also impaired by alcohol. The health of the liver may reflect on one's face—in the eyes or as a vertical line between the brows. These organs are also affected by a high degree of stress and trauma. It works both ways: high stress damages these organs and the stressed organ makes a person irritable and angry.

Similarly, the element 'metal' is connected to the lungs and large intestine. It is nourished by brown rice, and naturally pungent flavours like ginger, mustard, cloves, turmeric, wasabi and garlic. Root vegetables such as white radish and carrots also nourish the lungs and large intestines. The cheeks are associated with the lungs while the forehead and the lower lips are linked to the large intestine. The emotions connected to one's lungs and large intestines are grief and sadness. If one is sad for a prolonged period, their lungs are more prone to becoming weak. Similarly, if the lungs are already weak a person maybe more prone to sadness and grief. Again, it works both ways.

To sum up, macrobiotics is an understanding and awareness that can also be applied to diet. However, it isn't just a diet. It is an education where we constantly learn and refine our sensibility about the phenomenon that runs all of life. It is an understanding of the source and movement of energy around us: how we fit in as individuals into the environment, our body types, climate, age, thinking and consciousness, food etc. We can use this understanding to work towards our goals or towards a common purpose or universal cause.

Macrobiotics Is Not Japanese

Modern macrobiotics in the US has a Japanese influence, as the two original teachers and their wives were Japanese. One of them was Michio Kushi and his wife, Aveline Kushi. The other was Herman Aihara and his wife, Cornelia Aihara. Since their wives naturally knew more Japanese dishes, a lot of the original books and recipes by them have a Japanese influence. However, at the schools where I studied, they taught the universal principles in terms of nature and its five elements. They also taught us how to balance the masculine and feminine energies through lifestyle practices, work choices, life choices and food choices. They did not claim that nature could only be studied in a Japanese way. There is nothing specifically Japanese about connecting with nature or balancing the masculine and feminine energies. These are universal principles and should not be limited to any country or culture.

Many people often ask me, 'Why do people use miso (a fermented paste made from rice or barley and soybeans that aids digestion, blood purification and improves brain–gut health), shoyu (a high-quality fermented sauce) and tamari (a wheat-free soy sauce) in macrobiotics?'

Well, for one, this is because they have developed a taste for these. Second, most modern-day toxins are high in sugar, chemicals or poor-quality fat. They are acidic. All of these foods can be balanced with more alkaline, slightly salty foods that improve circulation, such as ginger and black pepper. Whether you wish to use miso, shoyu or tamari to balance the modern toxins, or use ginger, turmeric and black pepper, it does not matter. The idea is to understand the core energy-based principles of macrobiotics and continue to improve your understanding about how to best apply it to suit you. You can practice perfect macrobiotics without ever using miso, shoyu or tamari. These are not essential. However, if you have been exposed to the healing properties of these foods and wish to apply this knowledge to advance your health, then there is nothing wrong with that as well. The choice is 100 per cent yours.

The effect of food is beyond nutrients and calories. Simple nutrition is an incomplete view. Macrobiotics and Ayurveda, which are energy-based, are more valuable systems for a holistic approach to understanding and nourishing ourselves.

Macrobiotics and Asthma

According to macrobiotics, asthma is separated into two aspects. One is the actual attack and the other is the period between the attacks. The actual attack is a condition of 'excess' and the period in between is a 'deficient' state.

There are certain foods that create an excess in the body. Such foods have more fat and protein. For example, cheese is high in fat and protein. Even in its original and most natural form—as milk—cheese is a processed food product. Commercializing the production of cheese is probably one of the worst practices of industrialization. It isn't even a natural food after undergoing so much processing. Neither is it good for daily consumption. When a person eats cheese, their body gets more fat and protein than it needs. If the body cannot process this extra fat and protein, it begins to store this around the organs as visceral fat and as cholesterol in the blood. When this happens over a period of time, the body enters into a state of 'excess'. So an asthma attack is not something that happens in a moment. It builds over a period of days or weeks on an underlying energy level before any effect is visible.

Besides, the human body isn't designed to metabolize products high in fat and protein content such as cheese and ice cream. Some people have a very robust circulation and strong lungs that circulate and replenish chi (air) quickly. As a result, their recycle function is sturdy. They take in food, air and water and assimilate them while expelling unwanted toxins and fats quickly. These people may be able to digest high-fat and high-protein food a little better than someone with poor circulation and weak lungs. However, they cannot continue doing this forever. It may just take a longer amount of time before the cumulative effects are visible.

On the other hand, people with weak lungs and circulation may not be able to metabolize high-protein and heavy products like cheese and meat. These foods get stored as thick mucus in the lungs that ultimately block the air passages and bronchial tubes. The body is not able to break such dense fats down, which leads to the creation of mucus in the lungs and other pockets in the body. This depends on the quality and quantity of dairy or animal protein that is consumed. Soft dairy such as cheese and ice cream are usually stored in the upper body while hard dairy, eggs and meat are stored in the lower body, causing problems in the bladder or reproductive organs.

On the other hand, when the body does not get enough fibre, minerals or nutrients from wholegrains, beans, lentils and healthy vegetables, it is simply accumulating empty calories. If a person is not consuming enough healthy fats and proteins, his or her immune function and organ systems, including the respiratory system, could become deficient. This deficiency and weakness does not allow a person to improve their circulation and expel toxic matter.

Lungs Are an Organ of Elimination

Lungs, kidneys, large intestines and our skin are organs of elimination. When these do not function properly, the body doesn't expel excess acid and toxins. There is a certain amount of metabolic toxins that our bodies produce each day. Certain foods and meal combinations build more toxic matter in the body than others. The task of the organs of elimination is to remove the toxic air, fluids and other matter. If these organs are inflamed or blocked, then the toxins get stored in the body, causing blockages. Weak or blocked lungs, as in the case of asthma, are unable to remove toxins. This leads to the immune function deteriorating, leaving an individual more prone to allergies. This, in turn, weakens the lungs further and becomes a vicious cycle. This is why it is good to bring equal attention to eating healthy as well as eliminating and expelling toxins from the body on a daily basis.

2

Macrobiotic Practitioners vs Vegans vs Vegetarians

What is the difference between macrobiotic practitioners, vegans and vegetarians? Is one better than the others? These are important and pertinent questions people often ask. This chapter presents a few non-discriminatory observations and thoughts. As an author, my objective is to present unbiased, yet well-founded, views. As a reader, you have the freedom to adopt what works best for you.

Let's discuss this in three separate sections:

1. Macrobiotics
2. Veganism
3. Vegetarianism

Macrobiotics

The previous chapter outlined how macrobiotics is a comprehensive and profound understanding of nature's elements, food, cooking styles, our organs, and emotional and mental tendencies, and how it is all connected. It is seldom about the calories or vitamins. Even though a certain amount of calories are important for the body to function well, macrobiotics isn't limited to that alone. It involves a deeper awareness about the underlying energy systems.

Macrobiotics is plant-based. It is not necessarily plant exclusive. A macrobiotic diet isn't always vegan or vegetarian. The decision to adopt these diets is often made on the basis of genetics, health history, constitutional strength and current health. One doesn't have to be a vegetarian or vegan to follow the macrobiotic principles. We will discuss vegetarianism and veganism in detail later in this chapter. However, considering the aspect of a harmonious natural environment, many people prefer to not consume any animal foods. Hence, one can always be a vegan or vegetarian macrobiotic by choice.

Some people don't turn into complete vegetarians or vegans when practicing macrobiotics. Their nervous system is used to a certain amount of fat and protein. It is also related to the strength of certain energy channels in their body. Only if these channels are genetically strong and sustained with practices such as yoga and meditation can they completely give up all animal protein. I know of people who grew up on a diet rich in poultry and eggs and suddenly decided to turn vegan. Since they already had genetic weaknesses, it led to their nervous system being stripped off fat and protein very abruptly. This eventually led to them having many deficiencies as well as depression. Later, eating small amounts of fish wasn't enough for them to recover from the extreme deficiency. It took a comprehensive and well-thought out approach to help them get their energy and health back.

Each individual is different and so are their protein and fat needs. Some people may need a little extra fat and protein, while some may do fine with lesser protein consumption. To be able to absorb protein from beans, lentils and plant-based protein foods, one's digestion needs to be strong. If a person has a weak digestive system, they may find that eating even a small quantity of animal protein may boost the circulation and metabolic processes. On the other hand, some people may be able to build the digestive fire with home remedies, Ayurvedic medicines and/or a physical workout. The choice is yours. It depends on what feels better to your body, mind and values.

Every individual needs to educate and sensitize themselves about the principles of balance to ensure that they can build on strength in a sustainable manner. Without such self-education, they might cause imbalances that can take a long time to rectify. Hence, each individual needs a good counsellor when making big changes in their diet and lifestyle.

Veganism

It would be ideal to have a world of macrobiotic veganism. Such a world would be a euphoric era for humanity. In my opinion, in terms of individual energy and planetary health, it is the best practice to follow.

A vegan does not consume any products that come from an animal source. This includes edible and non-edible products. They don't consume honey or wear shoes or clothes that are made of leather or animal fur. The intention and integrity of such a thought process is noble and commendable. It reduces one's carbon footprint too, making it great from an environmental perspective as well.

However, some people follow a misinformed and distorted version of veganism. This can be quite dangerous as it can cause deficiencies. To sustain a vegan lifestyle, one must be up-to-date about all aspects of health. A smart vegan would include small quantities of grain, healthy and digestible forms of vegetarian protein, a large selection of vegetables and salads, fermented foods, healthy beverages, and alkalizing foods and supplements in his or her diet. They would also need an active lifestyle that works on the core of the body, that is, the abdomen. This would help sustain digestive warmth and healthy assimilation of the food eaten. A spiritual practice that sustains a positive outlook and mood, healthy relationships and a love for what they do are all important components of sustaining a healthy vegan lifestyle.

However, there are always exceptions that may require a different approach. Given my initial bias towards veganism, it makes me sad to admit that not everyone can easily follow a vegan way of life. Some people may need transition time to allow their bodies to prepare for it. Others may not be able to sustain it at all. The harsh reality contrasts my idealistic expectations. I have worked with and counselled people for over twelve years and had to change my bias towards veganism in certain cases to be able to get results. This has been a great learning experience for me. As a health advocate, I have to choose the best possible path for the person sitting in front of me instead of taking an emotional stand to not harm or eat animals. Macrobiotics has taught me to see the layers beyond a simple nutrition-based or vegan approach. Before I suggest something during a consultation, an individual's energy, genetics, past eating patterns, tendencies, deficiencies and other factors need to be taken into account. A macrobiotic counsellor is energy-sensitive and makes decisions based on the health of the person sitting in front of them. Sometimes, they may suggest limited amounts of animal protein to create an energetic and healthy balance for exceptional or transitional cases.

Vegetarianism

Vegetarianism is a little wider than veganism. Vegetarians do not consume animal meat but may have dairy products. Some vegetarians even include eggs in their diet.

A plant-based diet is always a healthy choice. Many cuisines in India have traditionally been plant-based. Our ancient wisdom and understanding has, in fact, inspired many people across the globe to lean towards vegetarianism. Culturally, Indians are passive and conservative. Eating animal foods leads to the creation of more active and aggressive energy and hence these foods have an adverse effect on the health, mentality, energy and personality of a person.

Modern-day processing and packaging brings into play many chemicals, antibiotics and hormonal injections. Eating animal foods today can affect the mind and body in a way that is worse than consuming small quantities from a natural source. In other words, an Indian who has eaten animal foods, especially commercial-quality processed meats and poultry, may have a tendency to have more mental, emotional and health problems.

However, I have seen purely vegetarian households suffer from health problems too. It is not enough for one to be vegetarian for only religious or sentimental reasons. An individual who has chosen a vegetarian lifestyle must avoid processed sugars, yeast, commercial-quality dairy, acidic drinks or snacks, and poor quality salts, oils and fats. Spending time to study energy-based nutrition and forms of exercise such as classical dance and yoga is also recommended. These forms of exercise help aid physical vitality.

From the perspective of increasing one's energy, you can opt for lentils. Generally speaking, individuals who consume lentils and beans on a regular basis have better health. We are lucky that the past generations grew up on a grain, lentil and vegetable palate. They didn't eat as much sugar, fried food and animal proteins as the new generation does. This is a cause for concern as the incidence of lifestyle diseases is increasing as a result. In fact, more cases of childhood diabetes and obesity are showing up now than ever. It is our responsibility to educate the present generation about the benefits of plant-based, chemical-free and home-made meals.

Golden Rules for People with Asthma

1. If you choose to eat animal proteins, eat it in limited quantities. It is preferable to have these in small quantities for a better energy balance. Supplement the meal with something light such as soups, salads or refreshing vegetable dishes. Even a little lemon, onion and/or grated white radish would be advisable to help digest the animal protein.

2. Make smart choices. An exclusive plant-based diet without any animal foods must be thought through in a very intelligent manner, perhaps with help from a macrobiotic or Ayurvedic counsellor, or an experienced doctor.

3. Simple sugars and vegan meat substitutes should not be consumed. Turning vegan and eating a lot of simple sugars and oils is not sustainable. Margarine is not a substitute either. A smart and sustainable vegan diet requires an intelligent approach with a certain amount of awareness and planning. For some people, being vegan is an emotional and ecological decision, and their efforts and stance are worthy of respect. However, they too must not neglect the principles of balance.

4. Choose organic products whenever possible. The amount
    of chemicals in the environment and food today is
    appalling. These chemicals are the main reason for many
    health deficiencies and aggravation of diseases.
5. Don't overdo eating raw foods and fruit. Raw foods and
    fruit are healthy additions to one's diet, but they shouldn't
    be the only thing you consume. It can work for people
    who have a lot of heat, or pitta, in their body. We must
    remember that fire is one of the five natural elements,
    which is why cooking using fire is essential for balancing
    all elements and sustaining long-term health and wellness.

3

Blood Sugar and Asthma

We consume food for energy. We need energy to perform our daily activities and to sustain the body and its functions (its cells, tissues, organs, muscles and brain).

Spikes and Crashes in Blood Sugar Levels Is Bad

Our body turns the food we eat into blood sugar. If the food we eat burns too quickly (like white sugar or refined flour), it gives us instant energy and satisfaction. Foods that burn quickly also spike or crash our blood sugar levels quickly. The spiking and crashing does not give the body steady energy. As the levels drop, so does energy. When such spikes and crashes of blood sugar levels happen over many years, they begin to affect one's emotional balance too. This also leads to spikes and crashes in one's emotional condition.

Whole Foods Do Not Cause Spikes and Crashes

One should eat food in its whole form, with its fibre, vitamins and minerals all intact, as they were grown and reaped. This takes the body longer to process, as a result of which the food is assimilated slowly. Most slow-burning foods also have a low glycaemix index, which release blood sugar and energy slowly into the body.

Blood Sugar Problems Are a Precursor to Other Issues

In macrobiotics, we see that most diseases arise from inconsistencies in blood sugar levels. Blood sugar problems are a precursor to most diseases in the body as it is through blood sugar that energy is released in our body. If energy is released in a 'spike and crash' way, our underlying energy will lack stability. If energy is released slowly and steadily, then it is more likely to be stable. This underlying energy is responsible for the functioning of our organ systems.

When blood sugar levels are erratic, all the cells in the body do not receive energy at the same time, or in time. Consequently, they lose their ability to perform in an optimal way. This means that the body becomes partially dysfunctional. Depending on an individual's tendencies, food and lifestyle choices, genetics, birth dispositions, environmental toxins, and stress etc., different people develop different health issues. Blood sugar inconsistency is the body's first alarm that something is not going right.

In many cases, the blood sugar levels are too insignificant to show up as a medical problem. Blood sugar tests can be deceptive and a blood sugar problem may not show in a medical report but a person may show symptoms such as the constant urge to eat, mood swings, fatigue, chronic exhaustion, memory problems and even depression.

The Relationship between Blood Sugar Levels and Asthma

With stable blood sugar levels and a good glycaemix index, nutrients and oxygen reach the deeper cells and tissues of the body. When the blood sugar levels are unstable, there is erratic supply of energy, oxygen and nutrients to the cells and tissues. If this happens often, then the circulation, metabolism and endocrine (hormonal) systems get affected. The stability of your body is at stake if the blood sugar levels are not stable. If that is the case, some parts of our organs, including the lungs, may not receive enough energy, nutrients and oxygen. With each passing day, this leads to an accumulation of toxic matter. In case of asthma patients, this usually happens in the innermost parts of the lungs and the bronchial tubes.

Blood sugar inconsistencies are a major contributor to the improper functioning of the lungs as well as the whole hormonal system. Slow-burning whole foods, anti-oxidant-rich foods, rejuvenating superfoods and foods that help improve circulation and immunity should be given priority for anyone who is on the path to healing.

4

The Relationship between Food and Inflammation

A person with asthma suffers from chronic inflammation of the air passages. Certain triggers cause the airways to become further swollen and inflamed. Thus, studying and understanding inflammation is essential to heal asthma. Like blood sugar, inflammation is also a precursor to many diseases.

According to the dictionary, inflammation is a 'localized physical condition in which a part of the body becomes reddened, swollen, hot and often painful, especially as a reaction to injury or infection'.

Now think about this, if the lungs are chronically reddened, swollen, hot, and painful, they are bound to react to intrinsic and extrinsic factors and triggers. When this reaction is intense, it manifests itself as wheezing, chronic coughing and shortness of breath, all of which together is called an asthma attack.

It must be noted that chronic 'reddened, swollen, hot and often painful' lungs and bronchial tubes are the key reasons behind an amplified reaction to triggers. To heal asthma, the first and most important step is to reduce inflammation of the respiratory system. Like blood sugar level inconsistency, inflammation also impacts endocrine and immune functions.

There are many things that cause and aggravate inflammation in the body. The four main contributors are:

1. Diet-induced inflammation.
2. Inflammation caused by exposure to toxic chemicals.
3. Inflammation caused by stress, abuse and/or lack of sleep.
4. Inflammation caused by lack of motivation and/or physical activity.

Diet-Induced Inflammation

One of the main causes of inflammation is a poor diet. When we consume food, it is processed in the mouth and stomach, from where it moves into the gut where it is eventually absorbed into the blood stream. The blood carries nutrient-rich food to all the cells, tissues and organs. Hence, in macrobiotics we look at the 'quality of blood' to heal any disease.

If a person has a diet rich in white sugar, refined flour, chemicals, preservative-laden processed products, commercial dairy, hydrogenated oils or any acidic foods, then their blood quality is likely to be weak. Weak blood quality opens up a person to infection and allergies. When someone tells a macrobiotic counsellor or educator about an allergy, the first thing the counsellor thinks of is the blood quality. If the quality is acidic, the person is likely to be more prone to infection, inflammation and allergies. If the blood is alkaline and mineral-rich, the person is more likely to be able to resist allergies. For example, before I came across macrobiotics, my blood quality was weak and deficient in minerals. So, if I ate tomatoes, eggplants and wheat flour at an Italian restaurant,

I would wake up the next morning feeling bloated, with light acne on my forehead or even cramps in my lower abdomen (a sign of inflammation in the gut). If I had two or three consecutive meals out, no matter how good the restaurant might be, I would experience bloating. But now if I have a meal with tomatoes and wheat flour, it has a milder impact on me, with lesser inflammation. This is a direct result of eating a balanced diet over the years. This is how a mineral-rich, highly alkaline diet can support a person suffering from inflammatory diseases such as asthma, bronchitis, arthritis, etc.

So which foods cause inflammation?

1. White sugar
2. Nightshade vegetables such as tomatoes, eggplants, bell peppers and potatoes (not including sweet potatoes)
3. Refined flour, especially commercially baked foods
4. Food colours and chemicals
5. Alcohol

This reminds me of a Chinese proverb that says 'whatsoever was the father of a disease, an ill diet was the mother.'

What Is a Healthy Diet?

1. 25 per cent is adding health-giving staple foods to one's diet.
2. 25 per cent is removing acidic, inflammatory and weakening foods from the diet.
3. 25 per cent is adding blood-cleansing, immunity-supporting, fermented and alkalizing superfoods.
4. 25 per cent is chewing well and eating with gratitude and joy.

How Can You Stay Healthy?

1. Adopt a daily diet consumed with awareness and guided by someone who understands the human system well.
2. Stay active and get at least one to two hours of exercise each day.
3. Be motivated and have a zest for work and life goals. Sometimes a bad work environment, no work or an unfulfilling career choice can weaken you and your health.
4. Ensure healthy relationships and a happy and stable home environment.
5. Try to live a consistent and orderly life (at least for basic daily activities).
6. Spend time in nature and engage in activities such as gardening, cooking, cleaning, bathing, walking, etc.
7. Wear and use natural items, cosmetics and household-cleaning products.
8. Try to enjoy a flourishing sense of community and oneness with universally progressive goals.
9. Take holidays.
10. Bathe in mineral-rich unpolluted water bodies such as lakes, hot springs and rivers.
11. Build core abdomen strength.
12. Try to let go of stressful memories and build happy ones.
13. Develop an authentic and deep understanding of energy, meditation, and natural systems such as yoga, macrobiotics, Ayurveda, tai chi, etc. This awareness opens up our horizons and freedom in terms of making choices.
14. Use your talents in a meaningful way.
15. Live your dreams and work towards your goals.

Inflammation Caused by Exposure to Toxic Chemicals

Certain industrial, environmental and home-cleaning products contain such heavy chemicals that even a little exposure can clog cells and tissues. Since these are synthetic and almost as tough as plastic, the body takes years to flush them out.

Even detergents and dish-washing soaps and liquids can irritate the digestive, nervous and immune systems. The inflammation caused by exposure to chemicals takes time to reverse with healthy eating alone. Sometimes, special detox, natural supplements and therapeutic massages are necessary to aid the cleansing of the body.

Inflammation Caused by Stress, Abuse and/or Lack of Sleep

Does inflammation cause stress? Or does stress cause inflammation? It is quite obvious that the former is correct. However, only people who have a clear and insightful understanding about the body–mind connection realize that the latter is also unquestionably true.

Stress Causes Inflammation

Macrobiotics recognizes that both our internal and external environments affect us continuously. If our internal organ systems are inflamed, then energy won't flow smoothly in our body and we won't be able to perform to the best of our ability. In such a state, we may perceive situations and things to be worse than our coping ability.

According to macrobiotics, the organs that are most affected by anxiety and stress are the heart, liver, spleen, lungs and kidneys. When one undergoes high stress, the blood flow to the liver is impeded, the adrenal glands produce excessive cortisol, and the heart (where the *shen*, or 'spirit' in Japanese, resides) becomes erratic and unstable. Blood circulation and digestion also get affected. It takes a lot of wisdom and mental peace to be able to overcome the chaos caused by external stress.

When our external environment isn't supportive, it affects our health, emotions and thinking ability. External stress or shock because of someone else's behaviour either freezes us or angers us. Either our energy is locked, or frozen, into the kidneys, or our anger disrupts the functioning of the liver.

If the stress stays for over a year, then the adrenal glands continuously produce cortisol to combat it. They work together with the kidneys and the liver to remove toxic matter from the body. If these organs become dysfunctional, then the body starts storing toxins, and energy and blood begin to stagnate. Continuous stress also represses the body's immunity, affecting its ability to heal. Prolonged stress severely affects digestion, assimilation and sexual drive. Safe to say that stress weakens an individual overall, leaving them unable to feel rejuvenated.

It is said that the spirit or the shen resides in the heart. So when a person is in an environment that is emotionally unkind or unsettling, it begins to affect their heart and blood circulation.

Severe stress, like abuse or trauma, can cause chronic inflammation. The symptoms described above can multiply by a thousand times depending on the level of abuse. Such damage may take years to reverse.

Restful Sleep

Night is when the body rejuvenates itself. It is while we sleep that the body undertakes repair work. We receive dynamic and pure universal energy in an uninterrupted form from the earth and sky. This energy heals and replenishes our body, mind and energy on a daily basis.

Lack of restful sleep is a person's worst enemy. If a person does not rest enough at night, the stress from each day builds up till the person's nerves, adrenal glands and kidneys begin to weaken.

Daytime is meant to be active while the night should be used to rest. That is when the immune system revitalizes itself. The shen[1] and the vital life force recharge at night and give an individual energy to last the day. If a person doesn't sleep well, he or she will constantly feel exhausted. This often begins to show as dark circles around the eyes, which is a sign of adrenal fatigue and kidneys weakening. This also shows up as tired looking skin, dry hair and poor posture.

Inflammation Caused by Lack of Physical Activity

Physical activity improves circulation and metabolism. It also helps improve one's ability to burn fat and flush toxins.

Even if we eat the best diet but live a sedentary life, the nutrients and oxygen will not circulate well enough to benefit us. A lack of physical activity leads to stagnation of blood and energy. Stagnation breeds acidity, inflammation and buildup of toxic matter.

---

[1] According to Traditional Chinese Medicine, shen refers to the 'state of consciousness', spirit, mental functions, vitality and presence.

Movement promotes health. With proper movement, there is circulation and an exchange of healthy fluids that leads to cellular rejuvenation and regeneration.

Besides daily exercise, the other ways to facilitate healthy circulation are massages, acupressure, warm towel rubs, loofah scrubs, ginger compresses, engaging in day-to-day activities and consuming a diet rich in leafy greens, and fermented and whole unprocessed foods.

The Vicious Cycle Between Food and Inflammation

5

The Top Five Food Causes of Asthma

Foods that cause inflammation, acidic reactions and mineral depletions, or are heavy in fat and those that can cause mucus, or weaken the immune function, are primary factors that contribute towards asthma or lung-related diseases. These are:

1. White sugar
2. Nightshade vegetables
3. Refined flour
4. Dairy
5. Food colours and chemicals

White Sugar

White sugar ingested directly or indirectly through aerated drinks, sodas, chocolates, candies, desserts, or any packaged and processed food is the leading cause of inflammation. Today there is enough medical research and evidence to establish the link between white sugar and inflammation. Some people are aware about this while others dismiss such information. I understand their apprehension to stop eating something that their body and mind have got used to, but giving up white sugar is a lot easier than it seems.

First, we must understand that it is the white, refined sugar that is bad and not the 'sweet' flavour itself. Many people equate discontinuing white sugar with quitting desserts. Sweetness is a part of the six healthy flavours; there is no need to give it up entirely.

To begin, replace white sugar with other forms of sugar such as dates, jaggery, palm sugar or organic raw sugar (which is between unprocessed jaggery and white sugar). The process of producing white sugar begins with a sugarcane (which one can chew), then moves on to jaggery and ends with raw sugar that becomes commercial, and often bleached, sugar. The latter should be avoided at all costs, especially by people with asthma or any other respiratory disorder.

Brown rice, or for that matter any wholegrain, in its original form is very nourishing. But when we remove the essential minerals and fibre from it, it is not as easily digestible.

Fibre and minerals aid metabolism. Without them, white sugar and refined flour are not fully or easily metabolized and end up as excess fat. In fact, excess white sugar gets stored in the liver and is deposited as fat.

Not only does white sugar not have minerals, but it 'steals' minerals from our body. White sugar is very acidic and creates an imbalance in pH levels. Our body needs a certain pH balance to function properly. The moment this balance is disturbed because of acidic foods such as white sugar, the body leeches minerals from bones and the nervous system. The body invariably finds a way to alkalize the blood again, even if it means taking away minerals from the bones, teeth and nerves to restore the pH balance. When the body's core systems such as the bones, teeth and nervous systems get affected, the immune system too is hit.

There is a reason behind the increase in the number of cases of osteoporosis and inflammatory diseases in the last few decades in many developed countries, especially India. People are consuming far more white sugar and refined flour than they did earlier. An increase in the quantity of one bad component brings down the quality of one's diet. Quantity itself makes a difference. So 'a little sugar' every day is causing a little harm each day. Did you know that one teaspoon of processed sugar is equal to a four-to-five foot sugarcane in terms of sugar content? The human body wasn't designed to consume so much sugarcane in one day, let alone in a few minutes as part of a cup of chai or snack. The concept of 'a little' for a person today is very different from what it used to be.

Often, people go by how their family, friends and society eat. Today, the increase in the names and kinds of diseases we see around is frightening. A society's or the mass's choices are certainly not the best examples to follow. Refining your daily choices with intelligence, awareness and observation, slowly and steadily, is better than following a herd mentality.

Fruits and Fruit Juices

Fruits are an essential part of a healthy diet. But given the weaknesses of our digestive and nervous systems, they should be consumed in moderation. Consuming a judicious amount of organic seasonal fruits is healthy, but too much can be harmful as fruits too are a source of sugar. When your body is weak and ailing, the intake of fruits and fruit juices should be limited. This is only temporary, until you regain your strength and vitality.

> Simple carbohydrates are made up of a number of sugar units that are absorbed into the blood immediately on contact with the mouth. Before you can say 'yum', it has already entered your blood and been distributed to the cells. This is where the problem begins. The change is so rapid that sufficient supplies of oxygen are not readily available to burn the sugar. This is why so-called alkaline fruits, in most cases, actually acidify the blood.
>
> —Verne Varona, author of
> *Nature's Cancer-Fighting Foods*

People who have a lot of fire, or pitta, in their bodies—or those who consume or have consumed large quantities of animal proteins in the past—can have a little more fruit than people who are not in the best of health. However, people with weak digestion or nervous function, mineral and protein depletion, a generally cold body, or a history of vegetarianism should be more careful about having too many fruits and fruit juices. This is not to say that don't have fruits, but limit your intake during recovery and periods of fragile health.

Fruit is very cooling and relaxing, but in excess can cause coldness in the body and poor circulation; nervous, erratic energy; and loss of sexual vitality. Juice is even more concentrated. Like monkeys and other primates that eat fruit as their main food, over intake of fruit and juice leads to chattering, mugging, and a mischievous nature. Irregular heartbeats, colds, excessive blinking, thinning hair in the front of the head, dandruff, high-pitched voice, weak lungs, rounded shoulders, stooped spine and a long, thin nose are characteristic signs of taking too much fruit and juice. Those who eat a lot of fruit tend to be taken advantage of by others.

—Michio Kushi and Alex Jack, authors of
The Macrobiotic Path to Total Health

Nightshade vegetables

Nightshade vegetables are part of the solanaceae plant family. These include tomatoes, potatoes (but not sweet potatoes and yam), sweet and hot peppers (but not black pepper) and eggplants. Tobacco and certain berries are also nightshade vegetables. Consuming such vegetables may contribute to acidity, inflammation, mineral depletion and disturbance of the digestive and nervous functions. They are also not good for people who have auto-immune disorders and food sensitivities.

These vegetables contain substances such as calcitriol and alkaloids. Calcitriol increases the amount of calcium in the blood and leeches calcium from the bones. Eating a lot of nightshade vegetables contributes to excessive calcium deposits in the tendons, kidneys and circulatory system. This interferes with the functioning of the immune system. Alkaloids have a drug-like relaxing effect on the body. There is a reason why potato chips and tomato ketchup, or extra tomatoes in curries, makes them delicious and relaxing. But such vegetables, in the long run, contribute to acidity, inflammation, nerve damage and mineral depletion.

Tomatoes, peppers and eggplants have a soft or hollow centre. This contributes to making the human core and abdomen, which is a very sensitive area, soft and weak. These vegetables also contain seeds which make the blood acidic. Even Ayurveda considers these vegetables to be toxic.

Nightshade vegetables are used on a daily basis in many households, sometimes as much as three to six helpings each day. Excessive consumption of these vegetables also contributes to inflammation in the lungs and respiratory tract. While small quantities may not affect a person, having them daily is detrimental to healing asthma or any other lung-related disease.

Sometimes people don't understand the impact of these vegetables unless they go off them completely for around two months. Reintroducing one of these vegetables after two months makes the impact clear. I find tomatoes, peppers and eggplants to be more harmful for people with asthma and respiratory disorders than potatoes. Of course, some of these vegetables may be used occasionally but are not recommended for daily or weekly use.

Refined Flour

Wholegrains like brown rice, millet, barley, etc., are intact in their original form. Cracked grains are broken down so that they become easier and faster to cook, like wheat dalia or barley dalia or millet sooji. Then there is grain flour, which we call atta. In fact, there is a wide variety of attas to choose from these days given the number of people who are sensitive to wheat and thus adopt a mix of ragi, brown rice, amaranth and chana atta. There is also pasta and couscous and other grain products. All these are generally good for consumption. Gluten-free pasta is easier to digest than the commonly available wheat pasta.

For a person suffering from asthma or any other respiratory disease, it is important to have at least one or two helpings of whole and cracked grains every day. They can also choose to have grain flour (atta) or a grain product once a day. Wheat-free noodles and atta are less harmful for anyone with digestive weaknesses and inflammatory issues/tendencies.

Commercial and Refined Flour Is Not Good

Commercial and refined white flours are harmful for health. Organic flours are better for daily use. For those who use it more than once a day, it is essential to switch to the organic version. Having bread and pastries regularly is extremely harmful. The addition of chemicals, preservatives, bleach or yeast to food products made from flour—or worse, from white flour—leads to them being one of the top ten foods people with asthma should avoid. White flour is pasty and sticky, and eventually becomes mucus. While chemicals and preservatives add to inflammation of the lungs, yeast burdens the metabolism and circulatory systems. All of these have a direct impact on one's lungs. Eating these kinds of foods, even once a week, can prove to be harmful for the respiratory system.

A Word about Bread

Commercial-quality bread and toast are not good for you either. They are made of white flour, chemicals and preservatives, and sugar and yeast. Such is the weakening effect on the lungs that these should be completely avoided by any asthmatic.

Sourdough bread made without yeast is a better option, but that too occasionally. Everything else either leads to the buildup of excess mucus in the lungs or leaves them weak.

The Bermuda Triangle

I find the combination of three food categories to be particularly regressive for lung health. These are white sugar, dairy foods and white flour. When these three are combined into one meal or one product, it is lethal. All three are sticky and pasty, and cause acidity and inflammation. Eaten together, they are a potential recipe for a bronchial or asthma attack. So the next time you visit a bakery to buy a pastry for yourself or your child, just think about the Bermuda triangle—white sugar, white flour and dairy.

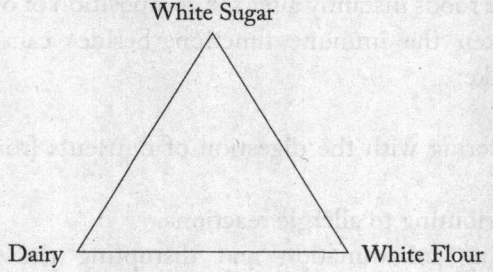

Dairy Products

Dairy products are a direct contributor to the production of mucus in the body. Mucus, in turn, is the leading cause of blockages in the lungs and respiratory system. Such buildup and blockage contributes to asthmatic symptoms and triggers an attack.

Food Colours and Chemicals

Synthetic or artificial food colours are the furthest you can get from nature and naturally grown foods. Any inflammatory condition can worsen in a matter of minutes thanks to these chemicals. In fact, food colours have been linked with hyperactivity, hives, itching, allergic reactions, tumours, inflammation, Attention Deficit Hyperactivity Disorder (ADHD) and even DNA damage.

Chemical substances are added to food to either enhance the taste and colour, or to ensure a longer shelf life. Sulphites, nitrates, tartrazine (a yellow food colour) and monosodium glutamate (MSG) often trigger allergic reactions. These are added to processed foods such as pickles, dried food, cured meats, canned foods, soy sauce, packaged fruit juices, packet soups, ketchup and fast food.

These foods instantly alter the composition of one's blood and weaken the immune function, besides causing other damage like:

1. Interfering with the digestion of nutrients from healthy food.
2. Contributing to allergic reactions.
3. Causing inflammation and disrupting the hormonal system.

If you suffer from any respiratory disease, you have to be more careful than others. It is advisable to stay away from packaged and processed foods. In case you do buy some of these, you must read the labels carefully. It is better to buy products from certified organic companies and genuine farmers' markets.

In Hindi, food colours and chemicals can be called asura foods. The word literally translates into 'out of tune'.

Fast Food and Restaurants

Fast foods tend to use low-quality salt, oils, soy sauce, yeast and chemical stimulants. Some Asian fast foods are probably the worst choice for your immunity and your lungs. You may not see an immediate reaction, but an attack doesn't happen overnight. Your lungs become weaker because of many reasons before it builds into a reaction and finally an attack. This doesn't mean that you cannot eat out, but that you must make more informed choices when you do.

Here are some tips you can put to use:

1. When eating out, choose cuisines such as south Indian, Thai, Mediterranean or Japanese, which are healthier.
2. The quality of the restaurant and its food are important.
3. Completely avoid fast-food restaurants.
4. Choose vegetable dishes that use the least amount of oil, sugar and dairy.
5. Choose dishes with quinoa, rice noodles, millet, sweet potato, rice, lentils, beans, etc.
6. For soups, choose barley, lentil, pumpkin, split pea or a vegan version.
7. Choose steamed, oil-free or light appetizers such as shumai, dim sums, sushi, fish tikka, salads, etc.

8. Avoid sugary and aerated drinks. Instead, choose small helpings of fresh fruit and vegetable juices or coconut water. Organic products are always preferable. Remember, quality makes a big difference, especially for someone with a weak immunity and asthma.

9. Chinese and pan-Asian food is one of the worst choices to make because it uses chemicals and MSG. Even if they claim not to use MSG, it simply means that they did not add it separately. However, a lot of the sauces they use already contain MSG and other chemicals.

10. If you choose north Indian or any regional Indian thali, avoid creamy, sugar-filled or oily dishes. Have a meal that includes millets or rice.

11. Order a side of steamed salad. If you are in a fine dining restaurant, order some raw salad to help digest the food better.

12. Avoid sugary or cream and dairy-based desserts.

13. Avoid poor-quality bread that contains preservatives and yeast.

14. Watch out for food colours and chemical-laden sauces and seasonings that are used in many Indian and Chinese restaurants. Don't choose dishes that are too red or orange, like tandoori dishes.

Finish your meals with herbal tea. You can choose from flavours such as ginger–lemon, jasmine and chamomile.

The Impact of Twenty Vices

If a person sticks to a healthy diet that includes fresh and whole ingredients, but occasionally has some organic packaged snack with small amounts of organic raw sugar, it wouldn't make much of a difference. It is the total impact of many wrong choices in one single day that creates an imbalance. If you add the few wrong choices from every day, the cumulative effect will be visible in terms of inflammation and immune function.

The collective impact of too many different wrong choices affects the body negatively. For example, if someone eats a little wheat, a little sugar, a little milk with tea, just one cup of coffee, a little bite of a dessert, a little overcooked vegetables, a few chips, a little yeast in bread, etc., all in one day, he or she might think that it was just a little bit. However, if you consider all of it, the end result will have an adverse impact on your blood quality and immune function.

Making the same wrong choice over and over again is also not good for the body. For example, having a bowl of chips everyday as an afternoon snack, or consuming yeast in bread every day is a bad option. Not only does it affect the immune system, but it also slows down metabolism and digestion that may lead to weight gain.

Too many wrong choices make the body give out warning signs in the form of an asthma attack or severe wheezing and coughing. Just the way that it takes a lot of uninformed choices to become unhealthy; it takes a lot of effort and healthy choices to reverse it.

Dietary Guidelines for an Asthmatic

Daily Foods	Weekly Foods	Occasional Foods (Once in 8–12 weeks)
Wholegrains	Rice pasta or gluten-free pasta	Deep-fried foods (home-made and using good-quality oil)
Cracked grains	Wholegrain pasta	Nightshade vegetables
Wholewheat and mixed grain chapatti	White rice (usually once or twice a week, if desired)	Alcohol (If desired, then grain-based drinks such as beer and rice wine are preferred)
Gluten-free chapatti	Sourdough bread (one or two times week if your health permits. Best if home-made.)	
Soup (in autumn and winter)		
Lentils		Any desired snack or food[1] (For example, vegan ice cream or a slice of vegan cake)
Beans	Soup (During spring and summer, soups may be consumed once or twice a week)	
Vegetables		

[1] What you eat once in a while is your choice. You can learn how these foods affect you and discontinue these as and when your desire for them goes away. It is the daily and weekly foods that need more attention.

Daily Foods	Weekly Foods	Occasional Foods (Once in 8–12 weeks)
Combination of blanched, boiled and raw salads Small quantities of organic seasonal fruits (During summer, you may consume a little every day or every other day) Fermented foods such as brine pickles, idlis, oil-free digestive lemon pickle, sauerkraut, pressed salads, etc. Sprouts and microgreens Almonds, walnuts, sesame seeds Warm or hot teas and brews without sugar or dairy Herbal supplements[3] as per your health and body type	Small quantities of seasonal fruits (During winter, fruits should not be consumed daily but only up to three times a week as per your health and body type) Sprouts and microgreens Sea vegetables, if desired Sugar-less and dairy-free desserts Fish[2] or your choice of animal protein (Generally, any animal protein should be limited to a maximum of three times a week, that too in very small quantities and if desired)	Sourdough white bread or white pasta

[2] Choose fresh fish according to what is clean and free of environmental toxins. Often, river fish is cleaner than seawater fish.
[3] Organic supplements as advised by your health counsellor and doctor.

6

The Relationship between the Quality of Fat and Asthma

A healthy diet typically includes unprocessed food and is low in fat content. It is the saturated fat that is bad, not the healthy fats. The body needs healthy fats in moderate quantities to store energy, insulate and protect vital organs, protect our nervous system and brain, maintain healthy muscle, keep our skin and hair soft and absorb fat-soluble vitamins and certain minerals.

Many people avoid fats to look thin, healthy and youthful. But when they see me or my friends in the macrobiotic community, they are surprised at how some of us can eat a lot of fat and still not gain weight. There is a reason why an energy-balancing approach is more accurate and effective than a calorie-balancing approach. We do need to pay some attention to calories and nutrition, but not at the cost of neglecting the energy balance.

To maximize the health of our lungs, a diet of low fat and low sugar is best for an easier exchange of gases. Aerobic activity increases the circulation within the lungs and helps keep its tissues elastic and resilient. Big offenders of lung tissue are the odors of chemical household cleaners, tobacco smoke (direct or second hand), carbonated drinks, excessive salt use, and alcohol.

—Verne Varona, author of
Nature's Cancer-Fighting Foods

To deal with asthma and respiratory diseases, we need to pay attention to three things that can help reduce blockages of the bronchial tubes and lungs:

1. The quality of fat.
2. The quantity of fat.
3. The production of phlegm in the body, and how and what leads to its production?

Quality of Fat

Let's examine food and the body in terms of lightness or density. Besides air and subtle energy/prana, the lightest thing we consume is water. Now, if we have a smoothie, it is slightly heavier than water but still very light. A banana milkshake is thicker and creamier. It is clear that the consistencies of water and banana milkshake are very different. The texture of the milkshake is closer to mucus than that of water or herbal tea. Similarly, mushroom soup with dairy cream and milk is more likely to trigger production of mucus in the body than a banana milkshake. Cheese is also high in fat and protein but without any fibre. It is much heavier than bananas, milk or cream.

If we eat a whole fruit, which is lighter, it gets digested and absorbed within 20–30 minutes. Vegetables have more fibre and are less sweet, which is why they are heavier than fruits, but are still considered relatively light. Salad leaves are lighter than ground and root vegetables. A gourd is also a light vegetable, while pumpkin is denser than a gourd. However, both are very nourishing and healthy. Sweet potatoes are denser than pumpkins. Someone who wants to reduce mucus and fat in the body should choose gourds and pumpkins, while someone who is skinny can have sweet potatoes more often. Though all three vegetables are healthy, sweet potatoes should be eaten in moderation. Grains, beans and pulses are heavier than vegetables and fruits. Despite their high-fibre, low-fat and high-mineral content, they are still light. Fish, meanwhile, is heavier than grains and beans, but much lighter than poultry and meat.

Vegetables and fruits hardly contribute to production of mucus, which is why they are easy to digest. Mucus produced because of dairy products makes the blood sluggish. It becomes sticky and is difficult to expel for the body. Mucus produced after consumption of excessive meat and poultry is harder to deal with.

A diet rich in cheese, poultry and meat is high in saturated fats and will contribute to thicker blood quality. If we consume sugar and refined pasta in addition to these high-saturated fats, our blood will become even more stickier and mucus-rich. This combination of high-saturated fats, refined flour and sugars leads to more blockages in the circulatory and respiratory systems, and could worsen an asthmatic's condition.

The relationship between saturated fats and heart diseases (and the circulatory system) is quite well established. However, the connection between saturated fats and asthma (and the respiratory system) is a relatively recent discovery. A research presented in 2010 at the American Thoracic Society International Conference in New Orleans suggested that individuals consuming a high-fat diet showed a higher airway inflammation. The high-fat diet also inhibited responses to the asthma-relieving medication. This research connecting fat and asthma has had a ground-breaking effect on the medical understanding of asthma across the world.

It is best to avoid a diet rich in saturated fats and refined sugar, as both lead to excessive mucus production and inflammation. Good-quality fats such as cold-pressed seed oils, nuts and seeds in their natural form, avocados, fish

(The text below is a summary of a study published by the American Thoracic Society on 17 May 2010)

People with asthma may be well-advised to avoid heavy, high-fat meals, according to new research. Individuals with asthma who consumed a high-fat meal showed increased airway inflammation just hours after the binge, according to Australian researchers who conducted the study. The high-fat meal also appeared to inhibit the response to asthma reliever medication, Ventolin (albuterol).

and natural fats in unprocessed foods are recommended in moderation.

Quantity of Fat

Moderation is often misunderstood or not practiced well. Even good fats should be consumed in moderation according to climate, age, occupation and lifestyle. If we are in a colder climate, we may need a little extra fat. In general, children need more fat and protein in their diet. Young people with an active occupation can also consume a little more fat and protein in their diet as compared to adults. Likewise, older people or people with sedentary lifestyles must limit their fat intake.

Production of Phlegm in the Body

The spleen is an important part of the immune system that works closely with the stomach and pancreas. It makes blood from food chi, ki or prana (life force) and is responsible for the transportation of bodily fluids. When the spleen is deficient, there is more undigested metabolic waste in the body. This creates an environment of dampness in the body, which means there is an excess of sluggish bodily fluids. As this undigested waste accumulates, it becomes phlegm and gets stored as fat. In Ayurveda, we refer to this as kapha dosha. A person with kapha dosha has excess mucus and fat in the body and is prone to sluggishness. There are many other connecting points between macrobiotics and Ayurveda as they are both based on an understanding of underlying energy.

Kidneys also play an important role in distributing and excreting bodily fluids. The bladder stores and excretes urine. If the kidneys lose their original energy and become deficient they fail to push forward waste to the bladder, making the excretory system weak. While spleen deficiency leads to the formation and storage of phlegm and fat in the body, poorly performing kidneys add to it by not excreting waste fluids.

It's important to note the quality of phlegm and fat accumulated in the body. Saturated fats lead to heavier phlegm and fat deposits in the respiratory tract, thereby leaving little room for air to flow in and out. Blockages are created if this continues for a while, leaving an individual prone to an asthma attack.

During an asthma attack, the muscles around the airways tighten. This makes it even more difficult for the air to pass through the already blocked bronchial tubes. Visible symptoms include coughing, wheezing and shortness of breath.

Here is a recap:

1. A diet rich in high fats such as dairy, meat and poultry, etc., makes the blood thicker because of more mucus.
2. Inflammatory foods such as white sugar, commercial and packaged foods, cheap-quality vinegar, etc., weaken the lungs, making them prone to an asthma attack.
3. A deficient spleen leads to more phlegm production, and mucus and fat accumulation that creates blockages in the body.
4. Deficient kidneys don't allow for healthy excretion thereby adding to accumulation of waste.

To control an asthma attack:

1. A diet should include less of bad and saturated fats.
2. A diet rich in anti-inflammatory and fermented foods is necessary. It's not just important to add these foods, but also to reduce the quantity of inflammatory foods.

3. If you are weak, it is necessary to temporarily reduce intake of fruits, at least till you regain strength and have stable blood sugar levels.

4. It is important to work towards improving the functioning of the spleen and kidneys. Improving blood sugar levels by including wholegrains and little or no refined foods is the way to improve spleen function. Processed foods are best avoided.

5. Energy-increasing exercises like yoga, tai chi and walking barefoot are beneficial for both the spleen and the kidneys.

7

Energetic Anatomy of the Lungs

A ccording to the ancient knowledge systems, lungs are the 'delicate organs'. They are the basic unit of the respiratory system whose primary function is to take in oxygen and release carbon dioxide. However, from an energetic perspective, they have many other functions that affect the whole body balance.

The health of your lungs is affected by your genetic health. Most core organs are formed while you are in the womb. Your mother's diet and health during pregnancy also plays a role in the genetic disposition of your lungs. In spite of genetic influences, the root cause of asthma and other respiratory diseases is diet, lifestyle, environmental toxins and stress. These triggers affect an asthmatic and can lead to attacks of a higher intensity if not managed well.

Since the lungs are very delicate and asthma is an advanced disease, it is critical to look at these four influences in detail. There is no space for ifs or partial attempts. For example, since asthma is ruled by chronic inflammation, you must remove all foods that cause inflammation from your diet. If you are serious about healing asthma, this has to be a priority.

Remember, half information will not give you desired results. Sadly, people who have scientific and medical information about a nutritional approach do not know much about how one's diet affects the lungs. They make a lot of effort and prepare a list of foods that they shouldn't eat. However, that list alone is not enough. It's like trying to clean your sweaty clothes with a vacuum cleaner. Similarly, a person eating without information about allergies will not be able to heal asthma or any other lung-related disease. We need to go beyond our understanding of allergies and nutrition, and look at the energetic anatomy of the lungs. While allergy information is viable and great, it is radically incomplete without an energetic understanding of lungs.

Energetic Associations for Lungs

Element: Metal

Partner organ: Large Intestine

Emotions associated: Sadness, worry and grief

Season: Fall/Autumn

Healing sound: Ssssssssssssssss (like the hissing of a snake)

Healing grain: Brown rice

Healing vegetables: Root vegetables such as carrot, white radish (also called mooli and daikon), burdock and kudzu root

Healing flavour: Pungent

Cooking method that helps: Pressure cooking (grains, not vegetables) and hearty stews

Associated facial feature: Nose, cheeks and part of the forehead

The respiratory and circulatory systems are closely connected. When a person has weak lungs, the life force (chi or prana) will not be able to adequately push blood. Often people with weak lungs tend to have cold hands. People with weak lungs also have weak circulation and get exhausted easily. Strong lungs indicate a strong circulation of blood. A powerful voice also indicates that the person has strong lungs.

Descending Function of the Lungs

Lungs are placed in the upper part of the body. From an energetic point of view, lungs have a descending action on the chi or prana. They direct the life force down to the kidneys which then hold it down to ensure the vital functions in the lower part of the body are in order.

There are two things that can increase congestion in the lungs. One is if the lungs are weak and do not direct the life force down. The second is when the kidneys do not hold the life force down. In that case, the energy moves back up to create congestion in the lungs. Also this affects how the kidneys and bladder perform. This is why congestion in the lungs and breathlessness may also be accompanied by water retention or urinary problems.

It is important to remember that both the lungs and kidneys are organs of elimination. If these are weak and partially dysfunctional, then the body will not eliminate toxins effectively, leaving the immune system compromised.

Also, according to Traditional Chinese Medicine (TCM), the lungs and kidneys work together to produce *weiqui*, which is also called the defensive *qui* (life force). If the lungs and kidneys are strong, then a person is able to get more nourishment from the food he or she eats. If the lungs and kidneys are weak, then a person is not able to extract enough energy from the food (even if it is nutritious).

Skin Texture and Lumps under the Skin

When an individual's lungs are weak, their face and skin often look dry or withered. When the lungs are strong and robust, the body receives and circulates oxygen freely, thereby giving one a fresh look. The lungs work together with the spleen to extract nutrients and prana from the food consumed. If the foods are more alkaline, refreshing and balanced, then the skin texture and tone is likely to be healthier.

When we eat foods that trigger the production of phlegm and fats, these get deposited in the lungs. Excess phlegm and fat goes into the skin, forming hard lumps. If excess phlegm and fat is formed because of consumption of sugar and dairy products, it may surface on the cheeks as pimples.

Understanding 'excess' is not rocket science. Wholegrains with beans, lentils, vegetables, fermented foods and some fruits are 'moderate'. Eating refined foods such as white sugar, white flour, dairy and too many animal products creates a condition of excess. This excess is pushed out of the body through different channels like the skin. In macrobiotics, the skin is known as the third kidney as it cleanses and detoxifies. Whatever is in excess in the blood shows on the skin.

Everything you eat becomes a part of your blood chemistry. Your white blood cells change every 14–21 days and your red blood cells change every 120 days. What you eat is partially absorbed and partially discharged through urination, faeces, sweat, breath and the skin.

When you visit a macrobiotic teacher or counsellor, they 'read' your body, skin and face. They reveal a lot about your health, lifestyle and what you eat. Your facial features, the colour of your skin, moles, blemishes, pimples, swelling, dryness lines and oiliness are indicators of your genetic health, current health condition and your blood quality.

According to TCM, the cheeks are indicative of how the lungs are. A puffy face, especially around the cheeks, hints at weak lungs. Vertical lines on the cheeks point to tightened chest muscles and restricted blood flow to the lungs. Freckles or brown patches on the cheeks indicate excessive intake of simple sugars. A cold tip of the nose represents weakness in the lungs and poor circulation. The shape of the nose is also indicative of one's respiratory and health tendencies. Swollen lower lips, which are quite common among many people who follow an unhealthy diet, are an indication of congested and weak large intestines.

Owing to long-term weaknesses and inflammation, the lungs lose their original elasticity and strength. Incidentally, a person with respiratory disorders may have a poor posture or a hunch, which further impacts the lungs as poor posture compresses them, leading to poor blood and air circulation. To improve the health of one's lungs, it is important to strengthen the abdomen and the core. Certain forms of Pilates (such as Stott Pilates), yoga, and breath work are particularly helpful in this regard.

According to TCM, certain organs work together and are called 'partner organs'. For lungs, the partner organ is the large intestine. If the lungs are weak, then the large intestine is affected too. Likewise, constipation hints at obstructed lungs. If both the lungs and large intestine are weak then a person may tend to sit in a way where they bend their knees and pull them in towards the chest, as if hugging the knees. This relaxes both the organs. People with weak lungs and large intestine may also feel the need to lie down more often than usual.

Grief: Emotion of the Lungs

The emotion associated with the lungs is sadness and grief and even worry. Worry and overthinking are also associated with the spleen. A person suffering from asthma and other respiratory diseases may tend to feel sad often.

An emotion can be the result or cause of a condition. If a person has been through a lot of sadness and lived in a bad environment, then their lungs become weak. It is important for us to not expose ourselves to ill-tempered people or high-stress environments, as these have a physiological impact on our lungs and the overall functioning of the body. Even medically, it is well established that stress is one of the major triggers of asthma.

Lungs are twin organs. Metaphysically twin organs indicate the aspect of dialogue of oneself with the outside world. The lungs, governing our throat and voice box, are all about speaking our truth and communication between the inside and outside world. Being mindful of our communication with others—or the lack thereof—as well as our internal 'dialogue' can be the first step in changing towards a healthier relationship with our body.

—Bettina Zumdick, teacher, counsellor,
author and humanitarian, and founder of
the Culinary Medicine School

Some people may feel fatigue while others may not be able to reduce their weight easily because of their long-drawn stressful environment. This happens because the respiratory system is closely related to the circulatory system. If the respiratory system is not functioning well, then the circulation of fresh oxygenated blood is hit. This may contribute to fatigue. Likewise, the three main organs that are impacted in case of an asthmatic are the lungs, spleen and kidneys. If all three are not performing optimally, then a person may not be able to lose weight. As we have read above, weak lungs may also contribute to dull, dry and pale skin, which can cause one to feel low, especially women.

In macrobiotics, we recognize that excessive emotions, abuse and stressful situations can lead to an imbalance. However, it must be noted that these emotions are also a healthy part of life, but only in moderation. New age slogans of 'Don't be angry' and 'Don't be sad, be happy' do not perpetuate an emotional balance. Every human being feels joy, anger, sadness, etc. These are important as long as one doesn't let them get out of control and keeps them in check in situations where they are not pertinent.

8

Seven Foods that Heal Asthma

The five elements in nature are associated with different organ systems, emotions, grains, etc. As shown in the diagram on the next page, metal (an element) and brown rice (a grain) are associated with the lungs, large intestine and skin.

Brown Rice

Brown rice should be a central part of the diet for someone who has asthma or any lung-related disease. If a person's digestion is weak, then it is essential to cook the brown rice in a way that makes it easily digestible. Softly cooked rice, khichdi or rice cream are good options. Initially, it can be eaten three to four times a week. For those who do not suffer from chronic digestive diseases such as irritable bowel syndrome (IBS) or ulcerative colitis, brown rice can be part of the daily diet.

Proteins to Nourish the Lungs

Horse gram lentils (kulath ki dal), brown chickpeas (kala chana), green and yellow moong lentils, black soybeans and adzuki beans are the five best beans that are good for the lungs. They strengthen digestion, kidneys and adrenal glands. This, in turn, fortifies all other organs. These should be well-cooked to aid absorption and assimilation. Also, they can be used in salads and the sprouts can be added to a hearty stew or soup.

Since the functioning of the lungs is closely connected to that of the large intestine, it is important to support the digestive process by cooking the beans well.

Pigeon pea lentil (arhar dal), mat bean (moth dal) and split chickpea lentil (chana dal) are also beneficial. Any bean which is dark in colour has a lot of minerals and doesn't cause flatulence or digestive discomfort is safe to be included in a healing diet. However, eating only refined or simple foods, like white rice, or refined dal is not healthy. People who eat only polished and refined dals may choose to do so if their digestion is weak. However, their want for ease in digestion

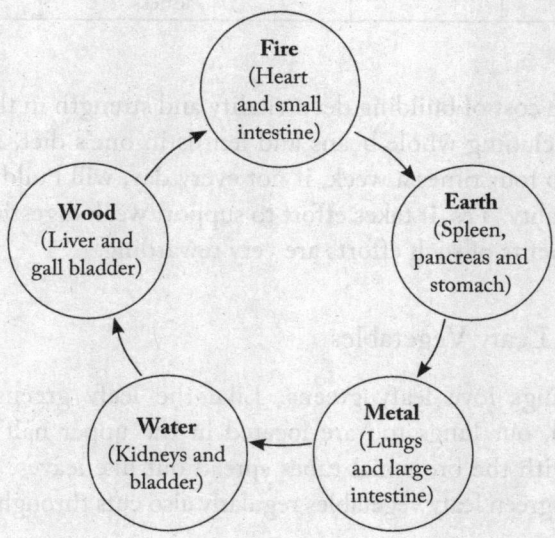

Theory of Five Elements

Element	Associated Organs	Opening	Associated Emotions	Taste
Water	Kidneys and bladder	Ears	Fear, courage will power, motivation	Salty
Wood	Liver and gall bladder	Eyes	Anger, frustration patience	Sour
Fire	Heart and small intestine	Tongue	Joyfulness, arrogance excitability	Bitter
Earth	Spleen, pancreas and stomach	Mouth	Empathy, jealousy worry	Sweet
Metal	Lungs and large intestine	Nose and Sinuses	Anxiety, confidence depression, sadness	Pungent

is at the cost of building deep vitality and strength in the long run. Including whole beans and lentils in one's diet, at least three to four times a week, if not every day, will build health and vitality. Yes, it takes effort to support weak digestion, but the benefits of such efforts are very rewarding.

Green Leafy Vegetables

The lungs love leafy greens. Like the leafy greens grow upward, our lungs too are located in the upper half of the body with the bronchial tubes spread out like leaves. Eating fibrous green leafy vegetables regularly also cuts through excess

Vegetables that help dissolve mucus	Vegetables that nourish the lungs	Vegetables that inflame the lungs
White radish with its greens	Carrots	Eggplants
Red radish with its greens	Pumpkin	Bell peppers
Lotus root/stem	Gourds: bottle gourd, snake gourd, bitter gourd, ridge gourd, zucchini, etc.	Tomatoes
Leeks	Amla	Potatoes
Scallions/Spring onions	Green beans	Hot peppers, except black pepper
Onions	Cabbage	
	Brussel sprouts	
	Cauliflower	
Ginger (in moderation)	Leafy greens: Goosefoot (bathua), fenugreek (methi), kale, collard, Swiss chard, spinach, watercress, dandelion	
Turmeric	Celery	
Mustard greens	Kohlrabi (also known as turnip cabbage)	
Broccoli	Therapeutic fresh herbs: coriander leaves/cilantro (dhania), Holy basil (tulsi), curry leaf basil, oregano, rosemary, sage, parsley, mint	
	All leafy green salads: arugula, rocket, lettuce, mixed salad leaves	
	Asparagus	

mucus buildup, which is partly responsible for an asthma attack. Reducing such buildup thus becomes important to keep an attack at bay. Consuming even small portions of leafy greens on a daily basis directly helps reduce buildup in the large intestine and lungs.

Mucus-Dissolving and Lung-Nourishing Vegetables

These include white radish, red radish, pumpkin, gourds, leeks, broccoli, cauliflower and sweet potatoes in moderation.

White or commercial brown bread, white pasta, cheese, butter, milk and sugar transform into mucus in the body. Pungent or bitter vegetables like white radishes, red radishes, turnips, leeks, ginger, spring onions (also known as scallions), bitter gourd, etc., help melt the mucus. Also, it is necessary to use calming, sweet and warm vegetables as well. Examples of these vegetables include carrots, cauliflower, cabbage, onions, pumpkin, sweet potatoes, etc. If you are trying to reduce excess mucus in your lungs and body, emphasize on pungent and bitter vegetables for the first four to five months, along with some sweet nourishing vegetables. Also include one to two helpings of leafy greens each day.

Fermented Foods

Trillions of microbes thrive in our gut. Not all of them are good. Our goal is to constantly increase the proportion of good bacteria. The winding structure of the gut resembles that of the brain. Energetically, they are both closely connected. In the medical and scientific world too, the gut–brain connection is much researched and talked about these days. The gut and brain are said to be connected by the vagus nerve. What we eat directly impacts our mental health and mood. This is not just a yogic understanding but is widely accepted in the medical world also. Many psychiatrists are in fact working with gut health to improve mental health. These days the gut is referred to as the 'second brain'.

Often, we have a gut feeling or a hunch about something. There is ample research suggesting that the vagus nerve carries messages between the gut and the brain, which establishes that there is a direct link between the two.

Foods that are fermented the traditional way with salt increase the proportion of good bacteria and microbes in the gut. This is not the same as fermentation in the case of beer or wine, or even that of old food left in the kitchen, which is basically rotting. Healthy ferments such as pickles, brine vegetables, sauerkraut, sourdough bread, kimchi, idli, dosa, appam, etc., give us good bacteria.

Sea Vegetables

Sea vegetables are not a part of many cultures. Nor does everyone have a taste for these. Sea vegetables are edible algae which are detoxifying and rich in fibre and minerals. They are good for the thyroid, hormones, nervous system and the bones. Here, it must be kept in mind that there are many ways to heal the body and mind as long as the healing paths are paved with awareness, intelligence and an understanding of your body type and constitution.

For those who wish to use sea vegetables, these are rich in calcium, iron, iodine, protein, vitamin A, B, C and E, potassium, zinc and other beneficial nutrients. These are also anti-inflammatory, beneficial for the immune system and particularly good for the thyroid, lungs, nervous system and the brain. You can refer to the recipes using sea vegetables in the international recipes section.

Sea vegetables that are particularly good for the lungs are wakame, nori and hijiki.

Sprouts and Microgreens

Sprouts and microgreens carry concentrated nutrition and should be a part of any healthy diet. Sprouts, which look like bronchioles, nourish their functioning and health. Sprouts and microgreens that should be used often include broccoli, fenugreek, radish, alfalfa, mustard, bok choy, sunflower, clover, green moong beans, mat beans and brown chickpeas.

Hot Cleansing and Warming Beverages

These include traditional hot teas from India and the Far East with healing ingredients such as ginger, turmeric, Holy basil, clove, black pepper, cinnamon, kudzu root, burdock root and lemon. The recipes for these teas follow in a later chapter.

9

Macrobiotic Home Remedies

This chapter includes recipes that are easy to make and include in your meal plan.

Ginger–Lemon Tea

Both ginger and lemon cut through excess mucus and fat. In the summer, have no more than half or one cup a day. During winter, you can have up to two cups a day.

The recipe below can serve 2–3 people.

Ingredients:

½ tbsp ginger, peeled and grated
1 cinnamon stick
3½ cups water
About ½–1 tsp lemon juice

Method:

1. Bring the grated ginger, cinnamon and water to a boil. Lower the flame and simmer for 5–7 minutes. Turn off the flame.
2. Strain and pour the tea into a cup and add the lemon juice. Drink hot.
3. You can save the rest for use later during the day or the next day.

Tips and Variations:

1. You can add wakame to the cup before pouring the tea into it. Let it sit for a minute before you drink it.

Lotus Root Tea

Lotus root tea is a traditional recipe from the Far East. The recipe below will serve 1 person.

Ingredients:

½ cup liquid from freshly squeezed grated lotus (about 2 lotus stems)
½ cup water
Pinch of sea salt

Method:

Place all the ingredients in a pot and bring to a gentle boil. Simmer for 2–3 minutes or until the liquid thickens and becomes slightly creamy.

Ame Kudzu Tea

Kudzu is a root vegetable that strengthens the lungs and large intestine. It also helps improve the functioning of the circulatory and nervous system.

This tea can be had twice a week or as guided by a macrobiotic counsellor. The recipe below will serve 1 person.

Ingredients:

1 cup water
1 tsp kudzu root starch, diluted in 2 tsp cold water
½–1 tsp powdered jaggery or brown rice syrup

Method:

1. Add the diluted kudzu root starch to the water and stir well. Bring to a gentle boil on a medium–low flame while stirring continuously. Cook until the kudzu root becomes translucent and begins to thicken. Turn off the flame.
2. Pour into a ceramic cup and add the jaggery. Drink warm or hot.

Burdock Tea

Ingredients:

1 tbsp dried burdock root
2½ cups water

Method:

1. Bring the burdock root and water to a boil. Simmer for 18–20 minutes. Strain and drink hot.

Ginger Compresses

Ginger compress is a remedy for increasing blood circulation and reducing the accumulation of toxins in the body.

Ingredients:

1–1½ cups grated ginger, tied in a muslin or cheese cloth (do not squeeze)
Large stainless steel pot filled with water
3 medium–large towels
Thick gloves

Method:

Bring the water to a rolling boil. Turn the flame off. Place the ginger (tied in the muslin/cheesecloth) in the water for five minutes and remove. Do not squeeze the ginger. Remove and store in an airtight container in the refrigerator for future use. Heat water in a smaller pot to add to the main pot as it cools down.

Ask the person receiving the compress to lie down on his or her stomach. Wear gloves, roll a towel and hold it up from the corners. Dip the centre of the towel into the hot liquid. Bring it out and wring to remove excess liquid, keeping the corner dry, and cover the pot. Place the wet towel on the person's back. Tap touch to check if the temperature is okay. Cover with a dry towel and wait till the skin turns pink. This is a sign that blood is rushing into the lower back and kidneys to remove blood stagnation. Repeat with the third towel, keeping the ends dry. Wring out the excess hot water and cover with a dry towel to maintain heat. Continue for fifteen minutes. Then ask the person to turn over and continue for another five minutes on the abdomen and five minutes on the chest.

After the compress, the person may dip their feet in the water for ten minutes and then rest. It is best to do this just before going to bed. Also, the person receiving these compresses should try to relax. Try not to have a conversation and maybe play some soft music. Use a ginger compress twice a week for two months. Stop and repeat after a few months as needed or under the guidance of a holistic or macrobiotic counsellor.

In Case of a Wheezing Attack:

The following should be used in keeping with a doctor's advice:

Hot organic apple juice: Serve warm, organic, unsweetened apple juice on a medium–low flame and give to keep a person calm in case of a wheezing attack.

Organic coffee: A small helping of organic coffee may be used occasionally to relax a wheezing attack. However, after following the dietary instructions in this book, one should not consume coffee, unless absolutely necessary, as it weakens the lungs in the long run. The coffee should be of high quality and preferably organic. This remedy should be used sparingly.

Ayurveda and Asthma

10

What Is Ayurveda?

Ayurveda is an ancient Indian system of natural medicine and preventive and curative healthcare. It is said to be a 5000-year-old system originating in the Atharva Veda. The Atharva Veda is part of a larger body of text known as the Vedas, which are the most revered and ancient scriptures in the Indian subcontinent. There are four Vedas: Rig Veda, Sama Veda, Yajur Veda and Atharva Veda.

Ayurveda, which finds a mention in the fourth Veda, is composed of two words: Ayur, which means life, and Veda, which means knowledge. Hence Ayurveda is popularly defined as 'the knowledge or natural science of life'.

Ayurveda has to do with diet, herbal concoctions, specialized massage treatments, and movement and breath therapy. Like macrobiotics, Ayurveda also emphasizes on one's connection with nature. The five elements—earth, water, fire, air and space—are studied and used in Ayurvedic healing. It also offers precise insight into how nature is connected to the human body. Energies present in nature are also present in us; we are not separate from nature. The energies which constantly balance our inner and outer environment are:

1. Movement (Vata)
2. Transformation (Pitta)
3. Structure (Kapha)

Each of us depends upon the balance between these three to function well. An imbalance leads to the digestive, metabolism, respiratory, circulatory, lymphatic and endocrine systems to work at a lower capacity.

For each person, at least one or two of these predominant energies is out of balance. Whatever is out of balance is called dosha, which literally means 'fault'. For example, if one has excess vata, it would be said that they have a vata dosha or a vata personality. This means that vata, or the function of movement in the body, is out of balance and not functioning at its best potential. Similarly, some people may have two doshas. The one which is more prominently out of balance is addressed first. Thus, if a person has a higher degree of vata imbalance and a lesser extent of pitta imbalance, then it would be said that they have a vata–pitta dosha.

Besides influencing health, these three doshas also influence the mind, personality and action ability of an individual. Vata is representative of the elements air and space. Pitta represents fire and water. Kapha represents earth and water. Air and space as elements are subtle and invisible compared to water, earth and fire. Hence, vata is a more subtle and invisible energy, while pitta and kapha are more physical.

11

Understanding Vata, Kapha, Pitta

Vata

Vata is subtle, yet has maximum influence on the well-being of a person. It manifests as the subtlest energy but still has the maximum control or influence. Vata is cold, light and dry, and represents movement. Since it is light (representing air and space), it moves very rapidly. Thus, vata dosha creates chaos in the body and mind.

When in excess, Vata affects the 'movement' or 'flow' between different parts of the body. In the mind, the chaos manifests as overthinking, over-imagining, and worried and rambling thoughts. In the body, it can be identified as dryness, poor digestion, flatulence, joint pain, intolerance to the cold or wind, a weak nervous system and even frigidity. Vata, however, varies from day to day.

Here is a list of tendencies for a person with vata dosha:

1. They have higher than usual intelligence and mental capabilities. However, their body may be fragile.
2. They may have a weak digestion and food sensitivities.

3. They may have dry skin. They may also be prone to dandruff.

4. They may feel stressed more easily. They may also feel emotionally down and exhausted.

5. The excess air and space element in their body is best balanced with healthy foods such as ghee, softly cooked rice, sweet potatoes, sweet berries, papaya, dates and pumpkin in small quantities.

6. Their anger rages quickly if they feel unheard or hurt, but it subsides soon enough. They don't hold a grudge.

7. They may have unstable blood sugar levels. It is advisable for them to eat slow-burning foods rather than quick absorbing foods like sugar, strong sweeteners, refined flour processed foods and coffee which increase 'quick energy' while they actually need more slow energy to balance the Vata.

8. They are more sensitive to the effects of chemicals as they have a weak nervous system. Hence, they should avoid packaged and processed foods. They should also reduce or avoid yeast in general.

9. They should avoid long gaps of not eating.

10. Vata is dry and cold, and hence they should avoid chips, crackers and baked foods.

11. They should generally keep themselves warm. Drinking warm water and hot herbal concoctions throughout the day is good for them. Likewise, they should avoid cold food and iced drinks.

12. They should not have too much raw food either. Raw cucumbers, lettuce and other light salad greens are tolerable for their digestion. However, they should avoid having raw broccoli, cauliflower, carrots and other hearty vegetables.

13. They should not follow food fads and must have a consistent and stable approach to their health regime.

14. Since vata is also dry and light, they should consume foods that are slightly heavy, sweet and moist. For example, sweet potatoes and dates pan-fried with a little ghee.

15. They usually have an elevated intuition and perception about spiritual matters. They also have a very delicate, subtle and refined taste.

16. They are often attracted to mind-over-matter theories. They may also be too idealistic.

17. A vata person should choose friends and mentors carefully. Cold and harsh people will drain them emotionally. Warm, sweet and nurturing people will help them bloom.

18. They get easily affected by loud noises. Since their nervous system is very open, they get affected by their surroundings very easily and sometimes have strong visual likes and dislikes. Since they are sensitive, they absorb both negatives and positives easily.

19. They should avoid or reduce intake of coffee. Even green tea should not be consumed on a daily basis. Green tea may be beneficial after a restaurant-style greasy meal or on days they consume animal protein.

20. A person with very high vata may like to live a life of service rather than a business-oriented life.

High stress, abuse or trauma can literally freeze a vata personality. The pain and emotions can go deep into their system causing chronic depression and pain. Their emotions dry out and they need more fire, warmth and passion. They may not be able to create the passion for themselves if they are in a high-vata induced depression, and therefore being in nurturing good company is very essential for a vata personality.

Pitta

Pitta is a dynamic and intense energy. When a person has a predominant pitta dosha, they usually have good digestion, metabolism and circulation. Often, pitta is the second predominant dosha for some people.

Pitta also represents transformative energy. It contributes to our digestive fire. So, if the pitta is in balance, the digestive fire is good and the body can expel toxins more easily. This explains how a lot of people can eat just about anything and still stay fit. In contrast, people with weaker digestive fire are affected by poor-quality food more easily.

According to Ayurveda, digestive fire plays a key role in healing many diseases. Hence having a balanced pitta is a desirable quality.

Here are the general tendencies for a person with a predominant pitta dosha:

1. They may have a reddish skin tone. They may also get rashes, skin infections and pimples more easily.
2. They generally have high intelligence and a distinct ability to process complex information.
3. They are often witty, smart and sharp.
4. They may have a tendency towards aggression, anger and intrusiveness. They may cross other people's boundaries without much thought.
5. On a physical level, healthy pitta shows up as good digestion, assimilation, circulation and elimination. Pitta is responsible for the conversion of food energy. If pitta

is low, then a person may have problems assimilating nutrients.

6. Their body gets heated more easily and they may sweat more than others.

7. They should consume cooling foods such as cucumbers, fresh fruits, raw salads, etc.

8. They should avoid very spicy or sharp flavours as this aggravates the pitta dosha.

Kapha

Kapha represents earth and water. It is more physical than the subtle energy of vata. Due its physical nature, kapha gives structure, stability and steadiness to the body. It gives the body a binding energy. Asthma is predominantly a kapha imbalance.

Kapha literally means water or mucus. Understanding the quality of mucus is the key to health.

It is common knowledge that human beings are 70 per cent water. Whatever we eat eventually becomes a part of the blood and lymphatic system. If one's bodily fluids or mucus are made from fat in wholegrains, vegetables or plant-based foods, one will have good kapha energy. Even bread and pasta form light mucus in the body. Consumed in moderation, say once or twice a month, they form light mucus. If had in excess, they can lead to sluggishness.

If the mucus is coming from sugar, it is stickier and causes more sluggishness. Sugar is also more acidic and causes more exhaustion. If the mucus is coming from cheese and butter, then it is thicker and may cause more fat deposits in different parts of the body. If the mucus is coming from poultry and meat, then it is even denser. Since animal protein comes from an active source, it also lends an active and aggressive energy to the body. This fights the sluggishness of softer mucus buildup. Excessive intake of animal proteins also builds up hard fats deposits in the body.

As per Ayurveda, the quality of kapha is very essential for improving health. It is important to understand kapha through the many kinds of mucus buildups in the system. In general, mucus from butter, cheese, sugar, refined flour makes the body weak. Also, if someone has more animal protein than what their body can assimilate easily, it could be regressive to their well-being. Remember, quantity controls quality.

The general tendencies for a person with a predominant kapha dosha are:

1. They usually have a stable and solid frame. They are sometimes heavier and may find it difficult to lose weight.
2. If kapha is predominant, their digestion is sluggish.
3. From an oriental perspective, they have more 'dampness' in their system. Kapha represents heavy, stable and moist energy.
4. They may be more attached to material things.
5. They may have more endurance, patience, gentleness and sweetness. If they are aggressive, they will likely be passive-aggressive.
6. They usually consume too much of sweet or refined food.
7. They take care of practical matters well.
8. They like to take care of family and friends.
9. Since they are more connected to the earth than spiritual matters (in contrast to vata that is more connected to ethereal and spiritual matters), they may be heavier.

10. They are usually more anchored and stable in their goals. Generally, these are positive qualities. However, if applied negatively, they may become tenacious.
11. They usually have smooth and well-hydrated skin.
12. Since Kapha is cold and heavy, they should avoid cold and heavy foods such as ice cream, aerated drinks and artificially sweetened foods.
13. They should also avoid greasy food and refined flour (especially maida) and white sugar.
14. Warm cinnamon and ginger-infused water is usually good for them.
15. They should keep themselves active to reduce sluggishness.
16. They may not have a very aggressive nature (unless they have a kapha–pitta dosha) but may be stubborn, forceful and strong-willed. They may also be possessive.
17. For the most part, they have a very sweet temperament.
18. They are generally stable and dependable. They like to help others.

12

Asthma Is Largely Attributed to Kapha Imbalance

Asthma is caused by an imbalance due to excessive mucus buildup in the respiratory tract. Inflammation and weakness only contribute to a quicker reaction. Ayurveda sees this excessive mucus buildup as a kapha imbalance. Though asthma is largely the result of a kapha imbalance, pitta and vata too are believed to be out of balance in such a case.

The degree and quality of Kapha and the body type of a person lead to the symptoms differing for each individual. As discussed in the previous chapter, butter, cheese, sugar, refined flour can lead to a soft mucus buildup and inflammation. Further, if a person consumes more animal protein than what their body can assimilate, the excess fat and protein develop into hard mucus in the respiratory tract. So, if you have asthma or any respiratory disorder, it is important to note the quality and quantity of animal protein that you have. The first step is to remove cheese, sugar and refined flour from the diet. Likewise, animal fats and protein should be reduced too.

Usually, a Kapha imbalance may be accompanied by extra weight. However, in the case of asthma and respiratory disorders, the individual may be thin or even skinny. This may happen due to a genetic and chronic weakness. It may also happen if you are consuming too much salt (which is rare in asthma patients) or poor-quality foods with excessive chemicals, sugars or hydrogenated oils and trans-fats. Chemicals and hydrogenated oils or trans-fats cause acidity and inflammation. They make the lungs weak and inflamed and more susceptible to an attack. When cooking, it is important not to let the oil smoke as this is not good for the lungs. Smoked oil is in fact carcinogenic.

The nature of animal protein is contractive. Excessive amounts of animal protein will always contribute to the worsening of an asthma attack because of contracted bronchial tubes. This is a very simple correlation, yet many people are unaware about the connection between the effect of a larger quantity of animal protein and the state of the bronchial tubes during an attack. Minimizing animal protein such as meat and poultry is the key to healing asthma. If one chooses to eat animal protein, they should reduce the quantity and frequency.

Poor-quality fats are difficult to digest, assimilate, circulate and eliminate. From the Ayurvedic perspective as well, a kapha imbalance suggests that the body has excess oiliness, dampness and coldness. This means that the body has already stored enough mucus and fat but does not have enough heat or digestive fire to burn them down. The nature of fat consumed is pivotal in reducing a kapha imbalance and healing asthma. Fat from natural, raw cold-pressed seeds and nuts is lighter and easier to digest, circulate and expel than fat from dairy or animal protein. Dairy leads to the weakening of the digestive fire and causes an excess of kapha in the stomach and digestive tract. The excess kapha begins in the stomach and moves into the lungs. To pacify it, the body needs warm nourishing food instead of cold foods. Here, warm and cold refers to both the temperature as well as *taseer* (in effect on the body).

Poor-quality fat also stores toxins or *ama*. Ama literally means 'undigested food leading to toxic matter'. It is the basis of all diseases and builds up in the system when poor-quality foods are consumed. It also builds up when there is a weak digestive fire or pitta, when there is inertia, depression, lack of enough physical activity, or stress. Ama also increases in the system due to environmental toxins and chemicals or preservatives in food products, cosmetics, mould, yeast and pollution.

13

Foods Detrimental for Asthma

According to Ayurveda, healing asthma requires reducing Kapha-inducing and tamasic foods. Kapha foods induce relaxation, but an excess triggers sluggishness and slows down metabolism and circulation. Tamasic foods are those which give rise to inertia, or dull and stagnant energy. For asthmatics it is even more critical to avoid such foods. They need foods with more fibre and minerals to cut through the energy of bloating, sluggishness and heaviness. Foods they should avoid are:

1. Cold foods and drinks
2. Dairy
3. Oily, greasy, fried foods
4. Refined and processed foods
5. White sugar
6. Stale foods
7. Foods with yeast or preservatives

Cold Foods and Drinks

Asthma is predominantly a kapha dosha state. To address this, an asthmatic must have warm foods that help improve the digestive fire. Since cold food and drinks put off the digestive fire, these foods aggravate the kapha dosha. For example, eating ice cream or having cold drinks, or even buttermilk, could aggravate coldness in the body and increase the Kapha dosha.

For asthmatics, it is necessary to avoid cold drinks or food straight out of the refrigerator. Instead, they must drink warm water and warm–hot herbal teas approximately half an hour or one hour after each meal. They must avoid drinking water with food as this will reduce the digestive fire.

If a person with a kapha dosha craves cold drinks and ice cream, then it means that their body has a lot of dormant heat. This heat can be reduced by consuming fewer animal foods and eating light salads, leafy greens and vegetables dishes on a daily basis. A person's natural cravings speak volumes about their inner energy and health.

Dairy

As noted earlier, asthma is a chronic condition where there is excess mucus in the lungs that blocks the airway passages. There are two causes for the formation of mucus in the stomach. One is eating food with high mucus content and the second is a weak digestive fire. The highest mucus-forming food are dairy products.

You or your child may not react to dairy products after consuming it once. But over a period of time, it leads to mucus buildup in the lungs. Coupled with other mucus-forming foods, this is a huge underlying cause of blockages in the bronchial tubes and lungs. Dairy products are the first thing that should be removed from your kitchen if you or a family member suffers from asthma or any other lung-related diseases.

Oily, Greasy and Fried Foods

Kapha dosha is heavy, oily, smooth, stable, cold and slow. A person with a kapha dosha, that is, an individual with asthma or a lung-related disease, will have a certain heavy quality. This may manifest as weight or dense emotions and complex thinking. They need extra effort and more support to become more active to create more warmth in the body for increased circulation and metabolic heat. Oily, greasy, heavy and fried foods add to their already dense dosha and hence work against them. If they consume heavy foods, they become enslaved to their bodies rather than gaining strength, mobility and freedom.

This doesn't mean that they should not have any oil or eat only boiled foods. It simply means that they must consume good-quality fats in moderation and avoid poor-quality fats. For example, refined corn, soy, safflower oil, hydrogenated or trans-fats, commercial fats in pickles, restaurant food, frozen foods and packaged foods are highly toxic. These foods don't move easily in the system of someone with a kapha dosha. When they consume such food, part of it gets converted into energy and part of it is stored in the body as mucus, fat and toxins. In the long run, these foods diminish the immune function and increase their sluggish nature.

Healthy kapha energy has a sweet, nurturing nature. In excess, it lends an enslaving, crouching and submissive quality to an individual. If left unattended for long, it can lead to a tenacious nature or excessive attachment to material things. Also, not speaking up for themselves and storing aggression silently builds mental and emotional toxicity.

Food doesn't only create a physical structure and immune function for human beings, but it also has a large impact on our mind, body, emotions, ability to make decisions and consciousness.

Kapha comprises the elements of water (jal) and earth (prithvi). Hence, it has the energy of structure (earth) and lubrication (water). We connect with the earth everyday through the food we consume (since food grows on the earth). Many people miss this direct connection. So, a plant-based diet (not necessarily a plant-exclusive diet) is good for someone with a kapha imbalance or someone with asthma.

Kapha imbalances (vikruti) are due to poor dietary habits, bad food combined with toxins, slow digestion and pent-up emotions. To balance kapha, one should avoid heavy, cold, oily and sweet foods. Add Ayurvedic spices to your diet such as ginger powder or pieces of the root itself, cinnamon powder or sticks, cloves, black peppercorns and turmeric. Exercise regularly and keep changing your routine. Make sure your diet is flavourful, with varied textures, and do not repeat the same foods every day.

Refined and Processed Foods

Whole foods are rich in fibre, nutrients and trace minerals. Refined foods have very few layers of fibre and minerals with only the starchy, fatty and 'bulk' part of the grain remaining. Eating the bulk, without the fibre and minerals, makes them partially indigestible, leaving behind undigested byproducts that are toxic and slow down digestion and metabolism.

There is a universal rule: What you eat becomes a part of your blood chemistry. Refined foods are indisputably fattier than whole foods. Some refined foods are also stickier than their whole counterparts. For example, white flour (made into dough) is stickier than the whole or cracked grain that it is made from. This means that it would have more mucus quality after it becomes a part of your blood chemistry. Similarly, refined white sugar is also fatty and sticky and is more mucus-causing than unrefined jaggery or whole sugarcane. In general, all refined foods contribute to more Kapha and mucus in the blood. Too much mucus is deposited in the lungs and bronchial tubes, which are an easy target.

We must take a moment to reflect. The food we eat becomes a part of our blood, which is circulated throughout the body. The blood carries nutrients and fresh oxygen to all the cells and tissues. It removes toxins and carbon dioxide from the body. If the blood itself has high mucus content, fat and cholesterol, it could lead to an excessive mucus buildup in and around the organs. This includes the lungs as well as other organs. If the blood is rich in fibre, nutrients and minerals, then there is less chance of a buildup. To reduce mucus in the body, it is imperative that the blood quality be nutrient-rich.

White Sugar

Besides lacking fibre and minerals, white sugar is also acidic and inflammatory. Both acidity and inflammation cause weakness in the lungs. So, sugar has three bad effects: excess sugar becomes fat and mucus in the liver, sugar causes inflammation, and sugar causes acidity which weakens the digestive fire. When food is not metabolized, it creates ama (toxic matter and mucus) in the body.

Many people think that not eating sugar is just about the calories. They would rather work hard at the gym to burn these. However, it is not just about that. Sugar works against the blood chemistry, digestion and immune function, leading to higher susceptibility to allergies, infections, skin eruptions and other reactions.

Stale Foods

Cooking transmutes food to make it more digestible and to make the nutrients more easily available for assimilation. When you have freshly cooked meals, they also pass on the fire energy that is used while cooking it. This helps our digestive fire as well. When food is put into the fridge, it loses a little value. When we reheat it, it may still provide the fibre and some nutrients, but it is not as healthy as a freshly cooked meal. Grains and slow-cooked dishes remain relatively healthy if they are consumed within twenty-four hours, but boiled or blanched vegetables and salads should be consumed fresh.

Stale food or a few days old food bought off the market shelf is seldom nourishing. It creates more toxins and acid buildup in the system. I would choose home-made leftovers up to a day and a half later over a meal full of acidic components and poor-quality oil from a commercial restaurant.

Food with Yeast and Certain Blue Cheeses

Yeast and mould directly hinder respiratory function. Yeast contaminates the bloodstream, clogs the organs and fogs the brain. There are two kinds of fermentation. One is because of salt, sourdough or healthy starters, which aid good bacteria in the gut. The other is when food rots or when it is fermented without salt, and often with sugar such as alcohol. This takes away the good bacteria from the gut.

To heal asthma, it is essential to increase good and health-giving bacteria in the gut by consuming more home-made fermented foods.

14

Ayurvedic Herbs and Home Remedies for Asthma

Home remedies are therapeutic concoctions made at home that help improve digestion and immunity along with relevant changes in one's daily food. A home remedy is usually aimed at a specific purpose such as reducing inflammation or strengthening the intestines or reducing fat and mucus, etc. A remedy preparation is effective when repeated a certain number of times per week for about 10–16 weeks. One should not do more than a total of two to four remedies at one time. To heal asthma, we need:

1. Foods that melt or pull out excess mucus from the respiratory tract and body.
2. Foods and herbs that strengthen the lungs.
3. Foods and herbs that reduce inflammation.
4. Foods and herbs that help improve circulation and the digestive fire.
5. Foods and herbs that strengthen and heal the kidneys.

Note: Since remedies are potent combinations, it is suggested that you use organic ingredients as far as possible for maximum benefits.

Cinnamon Clove Giloy Tea (for 2 cups)

You can have this four or five times a week or as recommended by a natural health counsellor.

Ingredients:

1–2 cinnamon sticks
3–4 cloves
1 small giloy stem, broken down into smaller pieces
½ tsp fennel seeds
A pinch of organic ground turmeric
1 freshly crushed black peppercorn or a tiny pinch of organic black peppercorn
3 cups of water

Method:

1. Bring all the ingredients, except the peppercorn, to a boil. Then lower the flame and simmer for about 7–10 minutes.
2. Add the crushed peppercorn and cook for another 30–60 seconds. Turn off the flame.
3. Strain the liquid. Drink hot.
4. You can choose to leave some of the tea on the stove or refrigerate it and drink another cup during the day or the next day.

Ginger–Turmeric Tea (for 2 cups)

You can have this up to three times a week or as recommended by a natural health counsellor.

Ingredients:

1 tsp freshly grated ginger root
1 tsp freshly grated turmeric root
½ tsp organic jaggery, or brown rice syrup, or honey
2–3 fresh tulsi (Holy basil) leaves
3 cups water

Method:

1. Bring the ginger root, turmeric root and water to a boil. Simmer for 10 minutes.
2. Rinse the tulsi leaves and place at the bottom of an empty cup. Pour the hot tea and add a natural sweetener of your choice. Mix well. If adding honey, do not add when the tea is boiling hot. Let it cool for a minute or two before you do so. Drink hot.

Coriander Seed Tea

The recipe below serves 1 person.

Ingredients:

1 tbsp coriander seeds
2 cups water

Method:

1. Bring all ingredients to a boil. Simmer for about 12 minutes.

Black Seed Oil Remedy

You can opt for this three times a week or as recommended by a natural health counsellor.

Mix ½ tsp black seed oil (kalonji oil) with one whole organic black peppercorn and a few drops of organic raw honey. Consume on an empty stomach or two hours after a meal. Have it at the same time every day.

Edible High-Grade Oregano Oil

You can also try 1–2 drops of edible therapeutic quality oregano oil with half a tsp of cold-pressed organic coconut oil. This can be done two to three times a week, once a day, or as prescribed by a natural health counsellor.

Note: I recommend doTERRA essential oils.

Bitter Gourd (Karela) and Honey Juice

Add ½–¾tsp organic raw honey to the juice from two to three medium-sized bitter gourds. Consume once or twice a week or as recommended by a natural health counsellor.

Amla and Turmeric Juice

Juice two Indian gooseberries (amlas) and add a one-inch piece of turmeric root. Add ½ tsp organic raw honey and drink four to five times a week.

Note: No more than three remedies should be followed at one given time unless guided by your natural health counsellor.

Recipes

15

Nourishing Soups

Cooking for healing requires proper knowledge, clear thinking, practice under guidance from experienced holistic teachers and presence of mind. The energy of the cook affects the health of the person consuming the food. The way you cook also has an impact on how it affects your energy.

About fourteen years ago, I was visiting a senior macrobiotic teacher, Mona Shwartz, in Dehradun. On my very first day, she sent me into the kitchen to cook with her chef, Naveen. She asked me to make steamed dumplings. I told her I had never made one and didn't know how to. She said Naveen would teach me. I made my first steamed dumpling and took it to her. She had a bite and said, 'Well, very nice, my dear, and very delicate too.' Then spotting the beginning of a tiny tear in one corner of the dumpling she added, 'and a little weak, but getting stronger.'

I was surprised! She wasn't talking about the dumpling but about me. I didn't know that I was being assessed. I was tired from my drive up the hills that morning and had taken on her request to make dumplings. She explained to me that despite having never made a dumpling, I did not make the corners

103

too thick as many people do even after years of practice. Also, she noted that it had just the right amount of filling, which to her was a sign of fine judgement and gentleness of spirit. I was thrilled to receive such compliments from her. I remembered the numerous times I had tasted thick corners in dumplings and samosas and instantly connected them to the energy of the chefs. I was quite amused with her detailed observation about my cooking skills. As I was there for a few days, she enjoyed many different dishes I made, even though I wasn't quite prepared to cook on that trip, leave alone being assessed! It was all unexpected. Each day, she explained about natural intuition and how a dish made a difference to the health of the person consuming it. Finer details count.

Luckily, besides studying at a few macrobiotic schools, I actually spent time with teachers, gaining hands-on knowledge. Another time, I spent an entire summer with three teachers in the Berkshires and learning with daily cooking. Once a teacher saw me sort the beans very delicately and said, 'Tarika, don't be afraid to discard the broken and bad beans.' The same day, he said, 'Don't be afraid to use salt either.' In his own way, he was trying to transform my delicate energy to a more courageous, focused and strong energy.

How one cooks, stirs, how much oil is used, how much the oil is heated, the ingredients, how much salt one uses, how a person puts a dish together, etc., is indicative of their health. On the same note, the way a person cooks impacts the health and energy of the person consuming the food.

As you go through this book, cook with the feeling that you want to create something nourishing and healing for yourself and your family. Learn from this book and see the resource section for online and in-person holistic courses in Ayurveda and macrobiotics to deepen your understanding about cooking and the energy of food. I would love to see you excel, grow and spread this way of life. Hopefully, we may get a chance to meet in person during one of my workshops or nature retreats!

Here are a few practical cooking tips to note:

1. Cook only in stainless steel, cast iron or ceramic pans. Use high-quality and heavy-based stainless steel pans. Avoid plastic handles. Le Creuset is a good brand for ceramic pans, as their pans are made of heavy pure cast iron covered with ceramics. Even if you get scratches in the pan over the years (which is difficult in a Le Crueset pan), the inside is still cast iron and not any toxic material like many ceramic pans available today. Ceramic coated pans from other brands are okay to use until they get deep scratches that will leech the toxic inner material into the food. Avoid all non-stick and aluminium pans as they leech toxins into the food.

2. Use mostly organic cold-pressed and unrefined oils. Organic cold-pressed sesame oil, organic mustard oil and organic ghee are recommended for regular use. You may also use organic cold-pressed coconut oil in moderation. Use olive oil only if you get the high-quality cold-pressed version. Do not use pure olive oil or pomace olive oil. You may occasionally use organic safflower oil though not refined or commercial quality safflower or sunflower oil. Rice bran oil may be used occasionally as well, though mostly only for high-heat cooking. Refined oils should be avoided. Avoid using soybean oil, canola or other refined oils.

3. Use only high-quality heavy-based stainless steel, wooden or bamboo spoons and ladles. Avoid plastic or rubber

handles for these. Studies have shown that lower quality stainless steel can be impure and even harmful.

4. Be careful when you heat oil. Do not let it smoke as it becomes carcinogenic. If your oil gets smoked, then it is advisable to throw it away, wash the pan and use fresh oil. This is tricky but very essential for your health and sustainable wellness.

5. When pressure cooking or boiling grains or beans, do not cook on a high flame continuously. After the first boil or pressure, lower the flame to the lowest mark and put a flame tamer at the bottom of the pan. Cook on the lowest flame for the recommended time. For your reference, here is what a flame tamer looks like:

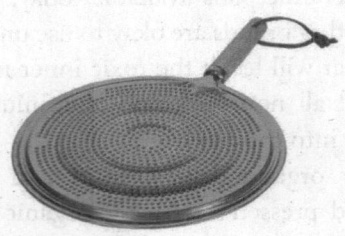

6. Eat at least one wholegrain dish per day and add at least one or two more wholegrain products (such as dalia or roti or home-fermented idli) into your diet. If you have weak digestion, limit the quantity of wholegrains or cook them very softly. Chew well, but do not avoid them altogether.

7. Do not use white sugar in the kitchen. If in India, use organic powdered jaggery, palm sugar (choose a high-quality, organic and dark-coloured version) or occasionally use desi khand. If you have the means, you may use high-grade maple syrup or organic raw honey occasionally. Do not use pancake syrup (that is what they often sell

when you ask for maple syrup) and use only high-quality pure maple syrup. Do not use honey where applying heat or cooking.

8. If using honey occasionally, use only raw honey. Also, use it in moderation as too much honey makes some people crave salty and baked food. It's not about the calories or superficial nutrition view but how this affects the energy, cravings and will power. Use organic raw honey in moderation in salad dressings where there are nuts and fibrous vegetables to slow down the blood sugar levels and help digest it. Avoid adding honey to boiling water or tea. You may, however, add it to warm teas.

9. Don't overdo any sweetener. Just because they are better than white sugar doesn't mean they are good for you. They should be used in moderation. Avoid having grains or beans with large amounts of natural sweeteners as the combination is bad for your gut.

10. For more healing benefits, use organic products as often as possible.

11. Eat plenty of leafy greens and salads. A person with asthma or any lung-related diseases must remember their helping of leafy greens every day.

12. Use tan and black sesame seeds often. Toast on a medium–low flame for 6–8 minutes. Let it cool down, store in a glass jar and sprinkle on dishes before serving. Also use ½–1 tsp of home-made black or tan sesame seed salt (page 196) every other day over rice or other grains. This helps improve lung function and bone health.

13. Always soak seeds overnight so that they sprout the next morning. Keep this rotation/habit alive. Use alfalfa seeds, fenugreek (methi) seeds, broccoli seeds, white radish seeds, moong beans, etc. Consume sprouts

and microgreens often. Grow sprouts at home using a sprout box and buy microgreens or learn how to make them.

14. Use plenty of fresh garnishes and leafy greens such as coriander leaves (cilantro), mint, basil, Holy basil (tulsi), curry leaf, parsley, chives, spring onions (scallions) often. These help improve lung function.

15. Eat home-made or high-quality dessert twice a week at the most. If you eat desserts often then the excess sugar may create bad bacteria in the gut, leading to many digestive problems.

16. Have soups often. In the winter, you can have it almost every day; in the fall and spring about three to four times a week; and in the summer at least twice a week. Consume pureed vegetables soups most often as these support digestion and immune function. Pureed vegetable soups also help relax the tightness in the chest and lungs.

17. Avoid plastic as much as possible in the kitchen. Don't use plastics to store hot food. Do not let plastic handles or utensils be close to the flame, especially a high flame, as the toxins from the burning plastic would clog the pores in a stubborn way, making the immune function weak and deficient. If plastic in the environment is non-biodegradable for hundreds of years, imagine how fumes inhaled from burning plastic in your own kitchen will affect your health? It will clog your insides and be difficult to get rid of. Beware of utensils with plastic handles and avoid high flames for such pots.

18. Let all fruit, salad greens and raw foods be 100 per cent organic.

19. Avoid all dairy products, except the occasional and moderate use of organic ghee.

20. Drink alkalizing and healthy warm beverages. Avoid sodas, aerated and sugary drinks.

21. Have fermented foods often. For example, sauerkraut, brine pickles, oil-less lemon pickle, other healthy pickles, pressed salad (also known as quick pickles), home-fermented idli, dosa, miso, etc.

22. Eat meals at the same time every day. Avoid late meals. Have breakfast between 8 and 9 a.m., lunch between 12 and 1.30 p.m., and dinner between 6.30 and 8 p.m.

23. Do not use a microwave. It creates an anti-spiral energy and chaotic digestion for the person consuming microwaved foods.

24. De-seed green chilies before using them. Use them sparingly if your condition is aggravated.

25. Reduce or avoid consumption of nightshade vegetables. If consuming tomatoes or bell peppers, make sure they are organic and de-seeded. Avoid eggplant. If using potatoes occasionally, make sure these are organic. Organic potatoes are a good source of healthy potassium, magnesium and zinc while inorganic potatoes may cause acidic reactions in the body and slow down healing.

26. Steam brown rice if you want to re-heat it. You can also stir fry leftover rice to make a new dish. Avoid re-heating rice in the same pan it was cooked in as this may lead to burnt bottom rice.

27. One cup of grain is usually good for four people while one cup of beans is also good for four people.

28. When making patties, tikkis, dosas, paranthas or pancakes in a large number, remember to keep a paper towel and a half-cut onion with you to wipe the skillet or pan to remove cooked oil every time you cook a new pancake, dosa, etc.

29. Use a timer when cooking rice or any grain or beans. This way you can take your mind off any worries about checking it and go about your other work in the kitchen!
30. Use wood or bamboo chopping boards. Avoid plastic.
31. To maintain a wooden cutting board, rinse and pat dry, and apply a little cold-pressed sesame or coconut oil to it once or twice a month. This will help prevent cracks. Also, avoid leaving the board in the sink while other dishes are being washed, as excessive exposure to running water may wop it.
32. Toast seeds and nuts in a larger quantity so that you can cool and store some in glass jars for use later. Planning like this can reduce cooking time on days that you have less time!

Our body is 70 per cent water, which is why our liquid intake has a critical influence on our blood chemistry and immune function. Every time we consume a healing, alkaline, therapeutic or curative drink, our stomach relaxes, the gut is cleansed and our kidneys receive essential support needed to improve the quality of our blood. According to TCM, the kidneys are the roots of life. They cleanse the blood and body and help restore mineral balance. So a healing soup or beverage should not be taken casually. It is vital to pay attention to every soup or beverage you have.

There are different kinds of soups that must be consumed in rotation to support a strong and healthy immune system.

A Nourishing, Pureed Vegetable Soup

A pureed vegetable soup is comforting and easy to digest. It is relaxing and nourishing at the same time. A healthy choice of vegetables would be a combination of root or ground vegetables. Green vegetables can also be used at times. However, root and naturally sweet vegetables are most nourishing. For example, you can choose a cinnamon–pumpkin soup, a pumpkin–sweet potato soup, leek–potato soup, cauliflower–cashew soup, broccoli–cauliflower soup, carrot–coconut soup, spinach soup or cauliflower soup. These soups should use natural oils and seasonings and nothing out of a bottle or packet. Pureed vegetable soups, when consumed regularly, naturally relax the body and are particularly good for those with a lung-related health problem.

In India, when I first say pureed vegetable soup to a student or client, the response I usually get is, 'Yes, I love pureed tomato soup.'

Hidden Vices: Tomatoes, Commercial-quality Sweet Corn or Mushroom Soups

Many people have a misconception that all soups are healthy. This isn't true. The quality and freshness of the ingredients make a big difference.

Tomatoes are considered to be a poisonous plant in nature-cure. Its leaves are regarded as poisonous in many cultures. Original Ayurvedic or Unani healing texts do not recommend acidic and sour flavours either. They consider the seeds of tomatoes to be particularly acidic and harmful. In fact, according to many cultures and systems of health, tomatoes fall under the category of nightshade vegetables. If you consume these, they are likely to interrupt your sleep cycle. Also, the acidic seeds may irritate your digestion and gut. Since it is hollow at the centre it is not good for our centre (the *hara*, our middle–lower abdomen area—the foundation of good health according to yoga, Ayurveda and macrobiotics). If the abdomen, which is also the core of our body, is strong and healthy, then the vital organs are protected. If this area is weak, there is often inflammation and impeded blood circulation that can lead to stagnation of blood and pain. Tomatoes are hollow with acidic seeds in the centre, which may lead to our centre becoming hollow and weak in turn. So, a pureed tomato soup is not healthy. People prone to allergies and inflammation should be particularly careful while consuming these foods. Tomatoes are also known to weaken the bones and aggravate joint pain. Since tomatoes are basically inflammatory, they aggravate symptoms of any disease whose name ends with 'itis'.

One man's food is another man's poison. Tomatoes serve a medicinal purpose for specific conditions. They might not work for people with asthma and lung diseases but are good for people with lower body stagnation and cancers such as prostate and ovarian cancer. People who eat a lot of meat and eggs are prone to diseases that affect the lower organs and stand to benefit from moderate consumption of high-quality organic tomatoes. However, even they need to be careful of too much use of tomatoes and must consume only organic tomatoes to reduce the effect of acidity on the blood.

Organic corn and sweet corn can be part of a healthy diet if they are grown naturally and are fresh. Having canned or genetically modified (GM) sweet corn, though very soft and sweet, is not a good option. Adding the brain-damaging MSG and other chemical-filled bottled sauces to a soup is certainly not healthy. In fact, it is so regressive that if this was the only soup being served at a party, I would rather not have soup that day. Sweet corn or other soups from a Chinese restaurant, or the two-minute packet soups that are full of neurotoxins and chemicals are sickness-causing. There is nothing healing or nourishing about them.

Mushrooms are high in protein content, even though some varieties are a little acidic. A creamy mushroom soup is a great addition to one's diet as long as it's not the only soup you have every day. Shiitake and maitake mushrooms, when consumed in moderation, are known to melt tumours in the body (under expert guidance of course). When consumed in excess, they pull away minerals from the bones and nervous system. Nobody should have more than two or three shiitake mushrooms per week.

Unfiltered Truth about Use of Tomatoes in Modern Indian Homes

Traditionally, tomatoes were used occasionally to add a delicious sour taste to food. Given the human desire to seek taste over health, some families started using them to please their family. They felt 'Wow! The dishes are appreciated more when more tomatoes are added.' Such thinking is so natural. Unfortunately, holistic information is lost to the modern housewife who doesn't know the side effects of daily consumption of tomatoes and how it affects the human physiology and mind.

Tomatoes are an example of how this tongue-satisfying, yet harmful, inflammatory vegetable has become so popular in every household that they are used almost on a daily basis. In fact, some people use it in multiple dishes every day. Such use of tomatoes without much care or awareness is at the expense of the health of one and one's family. Using lemon or tamarind is a better idea in comparison. Tomatoes should be limited to a maximum of three per week. If you are very weak, it would be advisable to avoid it completely for up to two to four months or until you gain strength.

If you have tomatoes and don't feel any side effects, then you have a strong digestive system. However, using lesser tomatoes will improve your health, even if its detrimental effects may not be apparent to you today. If, along with tomatoes, a person increases the use of other nightshade vegetables such as eggplant, potatoes and bell peppers, then they are creating more acid in the blood. Excessive tomatoes makes the blood acidic and the tongue gets used to the flavour, which is why people lose the ability to enjoy the natural taste of vegetables, all of which contributes to irritating the gut, leaches calcium from the bones, dilates the blood more than necessary (which is not good for people with low haemoglobin levels), increases inflammation and disperses concentration and focus for some people.

I love a little tomato in my diet, but I am aware of its effects on the body. In fact, I avoid it for a few months if I feel low on energy. One of my favourite foods is a tomato-based dish eaten with pan-fried bread. I also like cherry tomatoes or adding tomatoes to some bean dishes, or a condiment like peanut chutney. Tomato–kasundi pickle is the perfect addition to some meals. But would I choose to eat these every day? Or as much as Indian households do—that is two to four helpings every day? No. Never.

You can try this small experiment. Don't use tomatoes for two to three months to see how you feel. After that, resume occasional use.

Here's a little story to explain the effect tomatoes have on us. After a year or so of not eating tomatoes, I tried tomato pasta at an Italian restaurant. That was the first time I realized the effect it had on the body. People at the same table could not feel the effect as they consumed it regularly. Their blood had so much acid already that they could not tell the difference. In the last six months, I have eaten a lot more tomato on a weekly basis, as part of some vegetable or lentil. As a result, my blood carries the sour of tomatoes. Now if I eat a little tomato, I cannot feel the discomfort. It simply feels delicious and relaxing. If I repeat this, I begin to feel a certain amount of mineral depletion which shows up as a running nose or fatigue and even joint pain. Sometimes, it's not the tomato alone that affects my joints but it contributes to the pain along with the other foods that are not good for the joints. What I am trying to say is that when you are used to having tomatoes, you do not realize the negative effect it has. Leaving it out of your diet for a few months will help you assess how you feel with or without it.

Vegetable Broth or Clear Soups with Salt and Ginger

If you make a simple vegetable soup with fresh vegetables and a little ginger, it cleanses the body and helps maintain the digestive fire.

Grain-Based Soups

Grain-based soups are rich in fibre, vitamins, trace minerals and help you reduce weight too. They help regulate blood sugar, improve digestion and give you wholesome nourishment. Examples of such soups include pearl barley vegetable soup, barley–kidney bean soup, millet–sweet vegetable soup, soba in broth, pasta minestrone, rice soup or congee, etc.

Here is a list of soups you can choose from:

Chickpea–Leek Soup

Chickpeas help produce serotonin that relaxes the body and mind. They also nourish the pancreas and stomach. Since stress is a primary trigger for an asthma attack, this soup should be consumed often. Leeks are pungent and help melt excess mucus in the lungs and intestines.

This recipe serves 2–3 people.

Ingredients:

½ cup chickpeas, soaked overnight (you can discard the water in the morning), boiled or pressure-cooked until soft
2 cups leeks, cut in half lengthwise and then cut into thin diagonals
1 cup carrots, cut into small cubes or quarter-moons
½ cup pumpkin, cut into small cubes
2–3 cloves of garlic, pressed or minced
1 medium onion, cut small
1½ tsp cumin, ground
¼ tsp garam masala (optional)

¼ tsp turmeric
2 tsp organic cold-pressed olive oil or organic sesame oil
1 tsp organic ghee (optional)
Sea salt to taste
¼ cup fresh cilantro, stems removed and chopped finely
1 thin spring onion/scallion, cut thin for garnish

Method:

1. In a stainless steel pan, heat the oil and sauté the onions with a pinch of salt for about 1–2 minutes.
2. Add the pumpkin, turmeric and garlic, and sauté for another two minutes. Add a dash of water if needed.
3. Add the cumin and carrots with a little water. Cover and cook for 3–5 minutes on a low flame or until the vegetables are almost done.
4. Add two cups of water with the cooked chickpeas and stir well. Bring to a gentle boil, add the leeks, lower the flame and cook for another 5–7 minutes.
5. Add salt to taste and add 1 tsp of ghee. Cook for another 1–2 minutes. Turn off the heat, garnish and serve hot.

Broccoli–Cauliflower Soup

Broccoli and cauliflower, which resemble the alveoli, nourish our lungs.

The recipe below serves 2–3 people.

Ingredients:

1 cup broccoli florets

2 cups cauliflower florets
½ cup white part of leeks, cut fine
1 clove of garlic, minced or pressed
½ tsp sea salt, or to taste
1 tsp organic cold-pressed sesame or cold-pressed olive oil
1–2 tbsp spring onion/scallion or chives, cut small

Method:

1. Boil the broccoli and cauliflower with two cups of water and salt. Simmer for 7–10 minutes. Let it cool.
2. In a separate stainless steel or ceramic pan add the oil and garlic. Add the leeks and a pinch of salt, and sauté for two minutes. Turn off the heat. Let it cool.
3. Blend all the vegetables adding ½–¾ cup water to maintain the desired consistency. Keep the soup slightly creamy as it loses flavour if it is too watery.
4. Add salt to taste. Garnish and serve hot.

Tips and Variations:

1. You may add 1 tbsp sweet white miso and reduce the amount of salt accordingly.
2. Do not overcook after blending else the delicate flavour of the vegetables, sautéed leek and garlic will diminish.

Pumpkin–Sweet Potato Soup

This soup has a relaxing effect on the digestion, kidneys and the lungs. This is a very good option to help relax a constricted and stressed body and mind.

The recipe below serves 3–4 people.

Ingredients:

2 cups pumpkin, cut into small cubes
2 cups sweet potatoes, cut into cubes
1 cup leeks, cut fine
2 cloves of garlic, minced or pressed
½ tsp sea salt, or to taste
½ tsp organic cold-pressed sesame or cold-pressed olive oil
1-2 tbsp spring onions/scallion or chives, cut small

Method:

1. Boil the pumpkin and sweet potato with three cups of water and salt. Simmer for 7–10 minutes. Let it cool.
2. In a separate stainless steel or ceramic pan, add the oil and garlic. Add the leeks and a pinch of salt, and sauté for two minutes. Turn off the heat. Let it cool.
3. Blend all the vegetables to a creamy consistency. Add one to two tbsp of water as desired. Keep the consistency slightly creamy.
4. Adjust salt to taste. Garnish and serve hot.

Tips and Variations:

1. You may add 1 tbsp sweet white miso and reduce the amount of salt accordingly.
2. Do not overcook/heat after blending else the delicate flavour of the vegetables, sautéed leek and garlic will diminish.
3. If in a country other than India, you may use kabocha and Japanese yam.

Coconut–Lime Soup

Organic extra virgin coconut oil and milk are anti-fungal, anti-viral and anti-inflammatory foods. This is a delicately flavoured delicious soup that you can have with rice noodles too.

The recipe below serves 2–3 people.

Ingredients:

½ cup carrot, cut into quarter-moons
½ cup lotus stem, cut into quarter-moons
½ cup green beans, cut into 1.5-inch pieces diagonally
1 medium onion, cut into quarter-moons
¾ tsp sea salt, or to taste
3–4 cloves of garlic
¼ tsp fresh ginger juice
1 tsp lime or lemon juice
1–1¼ tsp powdered jaggery, or to taste
2–3 drops lemongrass oil (be careful not to over-season as the oil strengths vary as per different brands)
160 ml organic coconut milk (I use organic brands)
1 tsp organic extra virgin coconut oil
1–2 tbsp broccoli or alfalfa sprouts
1 tbsp fresh coriander/cilantro leaves

Method:

1. Heat oil in a stainless steel pot or wok and add the onions and garlic with ¼ tsp sea salt. Sauté for a minute.
2. Add the carrots and lotus stem, and a dash of water if needed. Sauté for 1–2 minutes. Add the green beans and continue to stir for another minute.

3. Add two cups of water and bring to a boil. Then lower the flame and simmer for 2–3 minutes. Add the coconut milk, 1 tsp of powdered jaggery and ½ tsp salt, and bring to another boil. Lower the flame.
4. At this stage, the soup is almost ready. The rest of the ingredients should be added just before serving.
5. When ready to serve, add the lemongrass oil, ginger juice and lime or lemon juice. Adjust the sweet and sour tastes as you like it.
6. Garnish and serve hot.

Spinach–Sweet Potato Soup

Both spinach and sweet potato help reduce bronchial sensitivity and improve lung function. The key is to use organic or naturally grown spinach as non-organic spinach can have unwanted side effects on digestion and immune function.

The recipe below serves 5–6 people.

Ingredients:

7 packed cups spinach (about 700 gms), rinsed thoroughly and roughly cut
2 cups sweet potatoes, cubed
3–4 cloves of garlic, pressed or minced
1 green chilli, de-seeded and cut small (optional)
½ tsp organic cold-pressed sesame oil
Sea salt to taste

Method:

1. Bring four cups of water to a boil. Add the sweet potatoes and ¼ tsp salt. Boil again and simmer for 10 minutes.

2. Add the spinach and cook for another 2–3 minutes on a low flame. Turn off the flame and let it cool. Sauté for 5–10 seconds.

3. In a separate stainless steel skillet, heat the oil and sauté the garlic for 5–10 seconds. Add a pinch of salt and the chilli. Sauté for another 30 seconds. Turn off the heat and add this mix to the vegetables. Blend and add ½ tsp sea salt or to taste. Serve hot.

Tips and Variations:

1. You may add ½–1 cup leeks or a little bit of fresh parsley for a refreshing change in flavour.

Creamy–Cauliflower Soup

Most white-coloured foods, such as cauliflower, white radish, leeks, white beans, etc., nourish the lungs and large intestines. This is a simple, yet delicious, and creamy soup.

The recipe below serves 2–3 people.

This soup is very simple to make and has been a success at many workshops and parties. It feels instantly nourishing. The trick is that this soup should be made and had fresh. If it is had cold or as a leftover, it loses its natural flavour and begins to taste bland.

Ingredients:

3 cups cauliflower
1 cup or 1 full leek, cut finely
⅛ cup cashews, soaked for 6–8 hours
½–¾ tsp salt, or to taste

½ tsp organic ghee (optional)
1 tbsp spring onions/scallions or chives, chopped fine for garnishing

Method:

1. Place the cauliflower in a stainless steel pot with enough water to cover them. Strain the cashews and add them to the pot. Add ½ a tsp of salt.
2. Bring to a boil and then simmer for 10 minutes. Let it cool. Blend until smooth and creamy. Add to the pot again and simmer. Add salt to taste.
3. Once it is warm–hot, add the organic ghee (optional), garnish with spring onions/scallions or chives and serve hot.

Tips and Variations:

1. You may add roasted garlic while blending the soup. Roast garlic in the oven with a little olive oil and a tiny pinch of salt until light brown.
2. You may add 1–2 tsp lemon zest just before serving for a summery soup. Use organic lemons when using the zest. Add the zest just before serving as boiling it may take away its freshness.
3. You can sauté the leek in ½ tsp sea salt with 1–2 cloves of garlic and add this to the cauliflower while blending. A little oil and garlic will add richness to the basic soup.

Barley Soup

Barley is known to melt dairy and animal fats in the body. It helps dissolve old hardened mucus in the lungs, kidneys and bladder too. Lemon is great for the liver. This soup is a must-have healing weekly addition in all kitchens!

The recipe below serves 2–3 people.

Ingredients:

⅓ cup pearl barley or ½ cup cracked barley (barley dalia), soaked in two cups water for 6–8 hours

2 shiitake mushrooms, rinsed well and soaked for 2–4 hours in a cup of water

½ cup or 1 medium onion, diced small

1–2 cloves of garlic, pressed or crushed

½ cup carrot, cut into small cubes

½ cup green beans

½ cup bottle gourd (lauki) or zucchini or cucumbers (peeled and de-seeded), cut into small cubes

1½–2 tsps sea salt, or to taste

1 tbsp high-grade cold-pressed olive oil (not pure or pomace olive oil)

Freshly ground black pepper, or to taste (optional)

2–3 tbsp cup fresh spring onions/scallions, cut thin for garnish

Method:

1. Heat oil in a ceramic or stainless steel pan. Add the onions and salt. Sauté on a medium–low heat for a minute.
2. Discard the stems of the mushrooms and dice small. Add the diced mushrooms and the soaking water and sauté for another two minutes.
3. Add the barley with its soaking water and another three cups of water. Bring to a boil and simmer on the

lowest flame for about 30 minutes or until the barley and mushrooms are cooked.

4. Bring back to a boil. Add the carrots and simmer for a minute. Add the beans and cook for another minute. Stir in the cubed gourd/zucchini/cucumbers, 1¼ tsp sea salt and ½ tsp of ground thyme. Simmer for 2–3 minutes. Adjust salt to taste.

Tips and Variations:

1. For a more Indian flavour, you can add cumin powder, coriander powder, organic ghee, a dash of lemon juice and fresh coriander/cilantro leaves.
2. You can also add leafy green vegetables to this soup. Leeks, white radish or sweet corn can also make for great additions.

Clear Broth Ginger Soup

This is a simple soup that helps dissolve mucus in the body. The recipe below serves 2 people.

Ingredients:

¼ cup pumpkin, cut into small cubes
¼ cup sweet potato, cut into small cubes
¼ cup lotus stem, cut into thin half-moons
¼ cup green beans
¼ cup broccoli florets
1 shiitake mushroom, soaked for 6–8 hours,
¾ tsp fresh ginger juice, squeezed from freshly grated ginger
1–2 tsp fresh lemon juice, or to taste

Salt to taste
4 cups water
2 tbsp fresh coriander/cilantro leaves, for garnishing
1–2 tbsp spring onions/scallions, for garnishing

Method:

1. Bring the water to a boil. Add the shiitake mushrooms after discarding the hard stems and cutting them into thin slices or small pieces. Lower the flame and cook for 20–25 minutes or till the mushrooms are almost cooked.
2. Bring to a boil again and add the pumpkin and sweet potatoes. Cook on a medium–low flame for 2–3 minutes. Add ¼ tsp sea salt and lower the flame. Add the lotus stems. Cook for another 3–4 minutes.
3. Add the broccoli and green beans and cook for another 1–2 minutes. Adjust salt to taste. Turn off the flame.
4. Just before serving, add the ginger juice, lemon juice, fresh coriander/cilantro leaves and spring onions/scallions.

Tips and Variations:

1. You may add a little organic tamari and noodles to this soup to make it an Asian-style noodle soup. Add salt accordingly. Omit the fresh coriander/cilantro and use more spring onions/scallions if you do this.
2. You may add some toasted sesame oil for added flavour.

Amaranth–Kidney Bean Soup

Amaranth was revered by the Aztecs as the food of immortality. Together with kidney beans, this soup is high in calcium and protein and benefits the whole immune system.

Amaranth is also known to reduce inflammation and cholesterol in the body. It is also good for people with anaemia and asthma.

The recipe below serves 4 people.

Ingredients:

¼ cup amaranth seeds
¼ cup kidney beans or pinto beans or runner beans, soaked overnight
1 bay leaf
½ cup carrot, cut into small cubes
½ cup sweet potatoes, cut into small cubes
1 tomato, de-seeded and chopped finely
1 medium onion, cut small
4 cups of water
1¼ tsp cumin, ground
½ tsp ground oregano
A small pinch of cinnamon
A small pinch of turmeric
A generous pinch of dried sweet basil
A pinch of black pepper
6 cloves of garlic, crushed or pressed
½ tsp organic ghee (optional)
1–1¼ tsp sea salt, or to taste
2 green chilies, de-seeded and cut small, or a pinch of red chili powder
1 tbsp organic cold-pressed sesame oil or cold-pressed olive oil or organic ghee
1 tbsp fresh coriander/cilantro leaves, for garnishing
1 tbsp spring onions or scallions, cut thin for garnishing

Method:

1. Place the amaranth, kidney or pinto beans, bay leaf, cloves and water in a pressure cooker. After the first whistle, lower the flame to the lowest. Place a flame tamer under the pressure cooker and simmer for about 45 minutes. Turn off the flame and let the pressure cooker cool.

2. Heat the oil or ghee in a stainless steel skillet. Add the cumin seeds, onions and a pinch of sea salt. Sauté for about 1–2 minutes. Add the garlic, chillies, turmeric, tomatoes and ¼ tsp sea salt. Sauté for another 1–2 minutes. Add a little water if needed.

3. Add the carrots, sweet potatoes and ¼ cup water. Bring to a gentle boil, then lower the flame and simmer for 7–10 minutes.

4. Once the beans are cooked, add the vegetables to the pressure cooker or a pot with the beans and mix well.

5. Season with ground cumin, oregano, dried sweet basil, pinch of cinnamon and black pepper. Simmer for about 5–7 minutes.

6. Stir in the ghee if you are using it and adjust salt to taste. Garnish and serve hot.

Tips and Variations:

1. You may add ⅛ cup organic sweet corn to this recipe.

2. You may add ½ cup shredded seitan (wheat meat) with 1½ tsp of organic taco seasoning to this soup for a Mexican flavour. Adjust salt accordingly.

3. If you want more beans, use ½ cup of beans.

16

Healing Wholegrain Dishes

Ancestral wisdom from all cultures centres meals around wholegrains. If you observe a plate from any culture and country, it will include rice, millets, wheat, corn, barley, buckwheat, oats, amaranth, quinoa, etc., as principal foods. Vegetables, protein dishes, salads, soups, pickles are an addition to these central grain dishes.

This may sound contradictory to many new fads that promote protein over carbohydrates. Sure, refined or quick carbohydrates may not be the best for you, but complex carbohydrates are necessary to restore the body's hormonal and blood sugar balance, and maintain strength. People who favour a high-protein diet must include small quantities of wholegrains. A diet with wholegrains is central to healing any disease.

If your digestion is weak, then:

1. For the first three months, eat wholegrains only twice or thrice a week. Gradually increase this as your digestion improves.

2. Make sure that the grains are soaked for 12–24 hours and are well-cooked so that they are softer and easier to digest.
3. Have plenty of pureed vegetable soups.
4. Avoid acidic foods that harm digestion, such as nightshade vegetables (tomatoes, potatoes, eggplant, bell peppers), white sugar, commercial-quality bread and dairy products.

Here are a few options you can try.

1. Pressure-Cooked Brown Rice (page 130)
2. Boiled Brown Rice (page 132)
3. Brown Rice Congee (page 132)
4. Soft Breakfast Barley (page 134)
5. Lung-Healing Khichdi (page 135)
6. Soft Millet with Sweet Vegetables (page 137)
7. Black Millet with Split Chickpea Lentils (bajra–chana dal khichdi) (page 138)
8. Millet and Vegetable Patties (tikkis) (page 139)
9. Pan-Fried Polenta (made with corn dalia) (page 141)
10. Fried Brown Rice (page 143)
11. Mona's Brown Rice Patties (page 144)
12. Red Rice and Foxtail Millet Idlis (page 145)
13. Soba Noodle Salad (page 147)
14. Brown Rice Salad (page 148)
15. Creamy Vegan Pasta (page 148)
16. Quinoa Lemon Rice (page 150)

Pressure-Cooked Brown Rice

Brown rice is one of the most important grains to help heal asthma and other respiratory disorders. Pressure-cooked brown rice is nourishing for everyone, especially for someone with weak lungs. Pressure-cooked rice should be made more in the autumn and winter while boiled rice should be had in spring and summer.

Rice is considered auspicious in many cultures. Brown rice gives slow-burning and steady energy to the body and mind, thereby balancing lifestyles and hormonal issues. However, some people are not able to digest brown rice easily. This doesn't mean that they shouldn't have it. All they need to do is to cook it softly and work on strengthening their core so that they can benefit from it.

The recipe below serves 4 people.

Ingredients:

1 cup brown rice, soaked in 2¼ cups of water overnight
1 pinch sea salt
Flame tamer (It allows for slow cooking for a longer period of time without burning the bottom. Slow cooking rice and beans has many long-term health benefits)
A timer
Bamboo rice paddle

Method:

1. Put the brown rice, water and a pinch of sea salt into a pressure cooker and bring to a pressure. After the first whistle, bring the flame to the lowest and place a flame tamer under the pressure cooker.
2. Cook for 45 minutes. Put a timer so that you don't think about the rice continuously.

3. Once cooked, turn off the flame and let it cool naturally. Rice keeps cooking in its own heat even after the pressure cooker is removed from the flame. This makes the rice softer and easier to digest. Once cooled, open and fluff the rice, turning the bamboo paddle. Mix the rice to ensure even texture. Serve hot.

4. If for some reason you are not serving it fresh, then you may steam heat it later. Re-heating in the cooking pot, in this case the pressure cooker, is not recommended as it would burn the bottom and make it more messy. Placing it in a steamer re-heats it evenly. Alternatively, since the rice takes less than an hour to make, you can place it in the pressure cooker and turn on the flame a little over an hour before you eat so that fresh hot rice is cooked and available when you want to have it.

Tips and Variations:

1. You may add some almonds, walnuts, lotus seeds or pecans to the rice before cooking to add a nutty flavour.

Boiled Brown Rice

Boil rice the same way as pressure-cooked rice. Bring the rice, water and a pinch of salt to a boil (instead of a pressure), then simmer on the lowest flame, placing a flame tamer below the pot for 45 minutes. Follow the other instructions, which remain the same as pressure-cooked brown rice.

Brown Rice Congee

The recipe below serves 2–3 people.

Ingredients:

½ cup brown rice, soaked overnight
1 medium onion, chopped fine
2–3 cloves garlic, pressed or minced
1 green chilli, de-seeded and cut small (optional)
1 small tomato, de-seeded and cut small (optional)
½ cup carrot or white radish, cut into small cubes
½ cup pumpkin, cut into small cubes
½ cup lotus root, halved lengthwise and cut into thin slices
1 bay leaf
1 tsp cumin seeds
1 tsp ground cumin
¼ tsp ground turmeric
1 tbsp ginger, minced
1 tsp sea salt, or to taste
2 tsp organic cold-pressed sesame oil
1 tsp organic ghee (optional)
2–3 tbsp fresh spring onions/scallions or fresh cilantro, cut small for garnishing
1–2 tbsp sesame seeds (toasted), or 1 tsp home-made sesame salt

Method:

1. Put the brown rice, bay leaf and a pinch of salt, along with the water they were soaked in into a pressure cooker. wait till one whistle. Lower the flame and simmer for 45 minutes. Turn off the flame and let it cool before opening the lid.
2. In a separate stainless steel or ceramic skillet, heat the oil and sauté cumin seeds for 30 seconds. Add the onions and

a pinch of salt, and sauté for 2–3 minutes. Add the diced tomato, garlic, green chilli and a pinch of salt, and sauté for another 2–3 minutes. Add the rest of the seasoning and vegetables one by one. Continue to stir and sauté. Add water as needed. Cover and simmer for 7–10 minutes. Set aside.
3. When the rice is ready, add it to the pressure cooker and stir well. Adjust salt and seasoning to taste and add a tsp of ghee if you wish to. Garnish and serve warm.

Tips and Variations:

1. You may add 2–3 black peppercorns before cooking, or ½ tsp freshly ground black pepper at the end. If your body is high in fire/pitta, or you have a lot of heat in the body and sweat a lot, then you should reduce intake of black pepper.

Soft Breakfast Barley

This recipe serves 2 people.

Ingredients:

½ cup barley, soaked overnight in 3 cups water
¼ cup carrots, cut into small cubes
2 tbsp green beans, cut small
¼ cup pumpkin, cut into small cubes
8–10 fresh curry leaves
¼ tsp salt, or to taste
½ small green chilli, de-seeded and cut small
1 tsp ginger, minced
½ tbsp organic cold-pressed sesame oil

Method:

1. Place the barley along with the soaking water and a pinch of salt into a stainless steel pot. Bring to a boil on a medium–high flame. After the first boil, lower the flame to the lowest, place a flame tamer under the pan and simmer for 30 minutes. Add the vegetables and cook for another 5–10 minutes.
2. In a separate stainless steel wok (kadai), heat the oil and add the ginger, green chilli and curry leaves. Sauté for a minute. Add the cooked barley to the wok and mix well. Simmer for another five minutes to let the flavours blend. Add water if needed.
3. Adjust seasoning to taste and serve hot with a home-made chutney of choice.

Tips and Variations:

1. You can make this dish with your choice of whole or cracked grain as breakfast. For example, you can use corn dalia, foxtail millet, barnyard millet, amaranth, etc.

Lung-Healing Khichdi

This recipe serves 2–3 people.

Ingredients:

½ cup short or medium-grain brown rice, soaked overnight
½ cup foxtail millet, barnyard or golden millets, soaked overnight (do not use ragi or bajra)
¼ cup Kulath dal (horse gram lentil), soaked overnight

¼ cup split green moong lentil, soaked overnight
2 cups pumpkin, cut into small cubes
½ cup white radish (mooli) or bottle gourd, cut into thin
half-moons or quarter-moons
1 medium or small onion, cut small
2 tsps organic, cold-pressed sesame oil
1 tsp organic ghee
1½ tbsp ginger, minced
1 bay leaf
1–2 cinnamon sticks
2–3 black whole peppercorns
1 tsp cumin seeds
¼ tsp turmeric powder
Sea salt to taste

For Garnishing:

½ tbsp toasted black sesame seeds
1 tsp home-made tan sesame salt
½–1 tbsp lightly toasted pumpkin seeds (if available)
½ tsp lightly roasted flax seeds
Freshly cut coriander/cilantro or parsley leaves

How to make:

1. Put the rice, millets, lentils, and five cups of water,
   cinnamon sticks, bay leaf, peppercorns and a pinch of sea
   salt into a stainless steel pressure cooker. After the first
   whistle, lower the flame to the lowest and place a flame
   tamer under the pressure cooker. Cook for 45 minutes.
   Let it cool naturally. Open and remove the cinnamon
   sticks and, if possible, the peppercorns.

2. In a separate large, stainless steel skillet or pan, heat the sesame oil and add the cumin seeds and ginger. Add the onion and a pinch of salt or turmeric after 15–20 seconds. Sauté for about a minute or two. Add the pumpkin with ¼ cup water and simmer for 2–3 minutes. Add the white radish and simmer for a few more minutes.

3. Once the vegetables are soft, add the rice–millet–lentil mix into the skillet and stir well. Adjust salt to taste. Garnish and serve hot.

Tips and Variations:

1. You can use this recipe to make amaranth, moong dal and pumpkin khichdi.

Soft Millet with Sweet Vegetables

Millet has a slightly drying effect on the body. Hence it helps pull out heavy mucus and fat from the body. I recommend having this dish once or twice a week.

Ingredients:

½ cup golden millets, or foxtail millets, or mixed Indian millets
5–6 cups water
½ cup organic carrots, chopped fine
½ cup organic pumpkin, chopped fine
½ cup organic cabbage, chopped fine
½ cup organic onions, chopped fine
1 green chilli, de-seeded and chopped fine (optional)
1 tbsp ginger, minced
1 tbsp turmeric root, minced (if in season)

Sea salt to taste

Method:

1. Bring the millets, water, ¼ tsp salt, ginger, turmeric and vegetables to a boil. Lower the flame to the lowest mark and place a flame tamer under the pot. Cook on low heat for about 15–20 minutes or until the vegetables are well-cooked.

2. Adjust salt to taste. Serve with home-made black or tan sesame salt and chutney of your choice.

Black Millet and Split Chickpea Lentils (Bajra–Chana Dal Khichdi)

This is a traditional Rajasthani dish.

One of the main causes of asthma is weak lungs and kidneys. When the body is cold, the kidneys are unable to hold down the energy from the lungs. Usually, the excess energy sent down to the kidneys is expelled through the bladder.

The black millets (bajra) and ginger used in this dish warm the body and help the kidneys maintain warmth, re-establishing normal functioning between the lungs and kidneys. This recipe is traditionally made with ghee that helps balance and absorb the minerals from the black millets.

This recipe serves 2–3 people.

Ingredients:

½ cup black millets, soaked overnight
½ cup split chickpea lentils, rinsed 3–4 times
½ cup bottle gourd, grated or cut into small cubes
1 medium onion, cut small

1 green chilli, de-seeded and thinly cut
2 tbsp ginger, minced
4–5 cloves or 2 tbsp garlic, minced
1½–2 tbsp organic clarified butter (ghee) or organic cold-pressed sesame oil
1¼–1½ tsp sea salt, or to taste
1 tbsp toasted black sesame seeds, for garnishing
1–2 tbsp fresh coriander/cilantro leaves, or spring onions/scallions, for garnishing

Method:

1. Put the water used to soak the millets, lentils and four more cups of water into a stainless steel pressure cooker. Add ¼ tsp sea salt. Bring to a pressure and then lower the flame. Cook for 10 minutes. Turn off the flame and allow it to cool for 30–45 minutes.
2. In a separate stainless steel skillet or wok, heat the ghee on a medium flame. Add the ginger, garlic and green chilli one after the other. Add the onions and ¼ tsp salt. Reduce the flame and sauté for a minute or two. Add the bottle gourd and sauté for another 1–2 minutes.
3. Add the millet–lentil mix and stir well. Adjust salt to taste. Garnish and serve hot.

Millet and Vegetable Tikkis

This is an easy and delicious way to include wholegrains into your diet regularly. Not only do millets help dry out excess mucus buildup in the lungs, but they also help improve digestion.

This recipe makes 12–14 medium to small patties.

Ingredients:

½ cup golden/cream/yellow millets (also known as foxtail millets, barnyard millets, sorghum, jhangora, samai, jowar, mixed white/yellow millets, thinai)

1¼–2 cups water (depends on the variety of millet used and the strength of the flame. Start with less and add more if required. For example, foxtail millets use more water than barnyard millets)

¼ cup carrots, minced

¼ cup celery, minced

½ cup or 1 medium onion, minced

1 tsp sea salt, or to taste

1 tsp cumin, ground

A pinch of ground thyme (optional)

1–2 tbsp cold-pressed sesame oil or organic ghee for pan-frying

½ cup sourdough bread crumbs or gram flour (besan) (optional)

Method:

1. Bring the millets with 1¾ cups water and a pinch of salt to a boil. Lower the flame and cook for 20–22 minutes or until the water dries up. Let it cool for an hour or two.

2. In a separate skillet, add 1 tsp of cold-pressed sesame oil and stir in the onions with ½ tsp sea salt. Cook for 1–2 minutes. Add a splash of water as required. Add the celery and cook for another minute or so. Stir in the ground cumin and thyme and cook on a low flame for another minute. Turn off the flame and let it cool.

3. When both the millets and vegetables have cooled down, mix the two and make 1.5-inch flat patties. Place these on

a plate and toss in bread crumbs or sprinkle some gram
flour on the top and bottom of the patties. Pan-fry until
golden brown.
4. Serve hot with cilantro–mango chutney or a chutney of
your choice.

Tips and Variations:

1. Pan-frying in ghee makes this dish more delicious. Also,
since millets are drying in nature, ghee adds the right kind
of fat to balance out the dryness for a person with high
vata.
2. You can use mashed potatoes or sweet potatoes instead
of the vegetables. These can be boiled and mashed and
added into the millets before making the patties. Adjust
salt and seasoning to taste.

Pan-Fried Polenta (made with corn dalia)

Polenta is made with cracked corn (corn dalia). Good-quality
corn is naturally sweet and has a relaxing effect on the body.
However, GM American sweet corn does the exact opposite.
So please don't use that in this recipe!

This recipe makes nine 2x2-inch squares.

Ingredients:

1 cup corn dalia
1½ tsp sea salt, or to taste
½–¾ tsp dried herbs of your choice (I used oregano and sweet
basil)
1½ tsp garlic, minced or crushed
Rice bran oil for frying

2 tbsp spring onions, scallions, chopped fine

Method:

1. Grind the corn dalia to make softer grits. (Usually, the version available in India is very hard and takes long to cook.)
2. Bring four cups of water to a boil. Add 1½ tsp sea salt to the water. Slowly add the corn grits and stir with a whisk to avoid lumps. Lower the flame and let it cook covered for about 20 minutes. Every few minutes, stir with a whisk to avoid lumps. Add another half cup of water, garlic and the herbs.
3. Continue to stir and cook on a low flame for another 10–15 minutes.
4. Once it is cooked and looks like a thick batter, pour it into a square glass container to let it set. After an hour, keep it in the fridge.
5. Bring it out after a few hours. Turn the square container upside down on a cutting board and cut the polenta into nine 2x2-inch squares.
6. Pan-fry in a cast iron or ceramic skillet with 3–4 tbsp oil. Cover the pan if the oil splutters because of the polenta's water content. Lightly brown both sides. Polenta is delicious when crispy but not burnt. Start pan-frying on a medium–high flame and then lower to lightly brown both sides. Garnish and serve hot.

Tips and Variations:

1. A cup of polenta takes anywhere between 4–5 cups of water to cook. More water than that may not set well. Keep it well-cooked and sticky thick before pouring into

the mould. If you add too much water, the oil may splash while frying. In that case, simply cover the pan.

2. Serve with herbed mushroom kudzu sauce or any home-made sauce of your choice.

3. You may also add a little umeboshi paste or umeboshi vinegar as seasoning just before serving.

Fried Brown Rice

Home-made fried brown rice is very healthy compared to restaurant-style fried rice. The quality of sauces used for commercial purposes are extremely harmful.

Even if restaurants claim not to use MSG directly, a lot of the bottled sauces they use already have MSG or similar chemicals that can damage the digestive system, brain and nervous systems. These toxic ingredients overstimulate the nervous system, weaken blood quality and contribute to free radicals and inflammation. All of this combines to make the lungs and immunity weaker, leaving an individual more prone to an asthma attack. An asthma attack builds over a period of time due to many reasons and has a final trigger. It's not as if the trigger is the only reason for the attack.

The variations of fried rice are endless. Here are a few examples:

1. Make Asian-style fried rice. Stir-fry cooked brown rice with ginger, garlic, onions/leeks, broccoli, carrots, mushrooms, lotus root, bok choy, green beans, sprouts and any other vegetables of your choice. Add a dash of organic tamari and lemon juice towards the end. You can also add toasted sesame seeds and cubed and pan-fried tofu.

2. Make jeera rice with jeera, ginger, garlic and vegetables of your choice in organic cold-pressed ghee or sesame oil.

3. Make tamarind rice with mustard seeds, curry leaves, minced ginger, de-seeded green chillies, vegetables of your choice, soaked tamarind and a dash of jaggery. You can use cold-pressed organic coconut oil.

4. To make lemon rice, you can add lemon instead of tamarind. Add roasted peanuts for added flavour.

5. To make summer spinach rice, you can use onions, carrots, spinach, garlic and olive oil.

6. You can also choose to make rice with winter greens, which is very therapeutic for the lungs. Make rice with mustard greens or radish greens. Add some garlic, minced ginger, onions/leeks, cumin and green chillies as desired. You can also add a dash of lemon juice and toasted sesame seeds just before serving.

Mona's Brown Rice Tikkis

This recipe is an easy and delicious way to introduce wholegrains to children and fussy eaters. Serve tikkis/croquettes with a sauce, dip or chutney that your family likes.

This recipe makes 20–25 small patties.

Ingredients:

3 cups cooked brown rice (1 cup uncooked)
1 medium onion, chopped fine and sautéed with a dash of oil and salt until golden brown
1 tsp ground mango powder
¾–1 tsp sea salt, or to taste
1 boiled potato, mashed (optional)

½ cup fresh cilantro leaves, chopped fine
2–3 green chillies, de-seeded and chopped fine
Breadcrumbs from sourdough unyeasted bread

Method:

1. Mix all the ingredients and make two-inch balls. Press to flatten them into flat tikkis.
2. Place breadcrumbs, with a little ground cumin, ground mango powder and salt on a plate. Coat the tikkis in the breadcrumbs and pan-fry on both sides until golden brown. Serve with a home-made chutney of your choice. It goes well with curry leaf chutney or coriander–mint chutney.

Red Rice and Foxtail Millet Idli

Idli is a fermented rice and lentil cake. Making this with wholegrains instead of white rice makes it more wholesome and nutritious. Fermented foods are good for our gut and blood. For a person suffering from asthma or any other lung-related disease, it is advisable to have home-made fermented grains like this for two to four meals per week.

Usually, idlis are served with a dip/chutney or sambar, a spiced lentil dish with lots of vegetables in it. If you do not have a taste for sambar, have it with any lentil or chutney of your choice.

This recipe serves 4–6 people.

Ingredients:

1 cup red rice, rinsed 2–3 times and soaked in two cups of water for 12 hours

½ cup foxtail millets, rinsed 2–3 times and then soaked in a cup of water for 12 hours

½ cup polished black gram lentils (urad dhuli dal), rinsed 4–5 times and soaked in a cup of water for 12–18 hours

½ cup red rice or flattened rice (poha)

1 tbsp fenugreek seeds, rinsed and soaked in 3 tbsp water for 12 hours

About 2 tsp of sea salt

Method:

1. Soak the grains and lentils as mentioned above.
2. Soak the flattened rice for 30 minutes.
3. After 12 hours, separately grind all the grains and lentils to a smooth consistency. This should be slightly thicker than pancake consistency.
4. You can mix the rice, millets, fenugreek seeds and flattened rice in one bowl and add ½ tsp salt.
5. Add ½ tsp salt to the lentil batter. Use a non-reactive bowl (I prefer a glass bowl). Cover with a bamboo mat or stainless steel sieve and let these ferment for 12–16 hours.
6. If you are in a place with hot climate, you can put them in the fridge after 12–13 hours. You can make the idlis now or keep the batter in the fridge for another 10–12 hours.
7. Lightly oil the idli moulds. Use only stainless steel moulds and not the plastic ones. Add water to the base of the pot in which the moulds will be placed for steaming. Steam for 20 minutes. Turn off the flame and let these cool for before removing. Serve hot with coconut or cilantro–mint chutney. You can also serve it with peanut curry leaf podi (ground seasoned condiment).

Tips and Variations:

If the idlis are hard, add a little more poha to make them softer. Also, they are dense as they contain more fibre and nutrition, and it's better to eat less grain which is more dense than a larger quantity of refined grain.

Alternately, you can use ragi (finger millets) to make the idlis. Use ¾ cup white rice flour, ½ cup ragi flour soaked overnight in a cup of water, a tsp of sea salt, ½ cup polished black gram lentil (urad dhuli) soaked in ¾ cup water and ¼ tsp sea salt overnight, 1 tbsp fenugreek seeds soaked in 3 tbsp water overnight. In the morning, add 1½ tbsp minced ginger to the lentil and grind till smooth. Add the ragi and rice flour mix and steam in an oiled idli maker.

Soba Noodle Salad

Soba noodles are made of buckwheat which has a drying effect on the body and hence pulls out mucus. Buckwheat is also good for the kidneys. I recommend using it once or twice a week at the most.

This recipe serves 4–5 people.

Ingredients:

2 bundles soba (about 200 gm)
1 cup snap peas, cut on a diagonal into 3 pieces each
¾ cup carrots, halved lengthwise and sliced into thin half-moons
1 cup lotus root, halved lengthwise and then sliced into thin half-moons
½ cup broccoli or radish sprouts

1 avocado, sliced thin for garnishing
2–3 tbsp spring onions/scallions, for garnishing and mix before serving, cut thin
2 tbsp toasted tan sesame seeds, for garnishing

For the dressing:

2 tbsp toasted sesame oil
2 tbsp raw honey, or high-grade maple syrup, or powdered jaggery, or to taste
2½ tbsp fresh lemon juice
1 tsp rice vinegar
½–¾ tsp sea salt or organic tamari to taste

Brown Rice Salad

Cooking should change as per the season. Summer cooking should be lighter, with more refreshing and citrus flavours while winter cooking should be a mix of light and hearty stews and dishes. Add steamed and raw vegetables of your choice to boiled rice, add coriander/parsley/mint leaves to taste and drizzle with a dressing of your choice. A light olive or toasted sesame oil dressing goes well with brown rice salad. You can also make it with caramelized onions, toasted peanuts, tamarind/lemon juice.

Creamy Vegan Pasta

This is a healthy replacement for cheesy mushroom pasta. For people with lung-related diseases, it is essential to avoid dairy products, especially cheese and cream, from their diet.

This recipe serves 2–3 people.

Ingredients:

200 gm gluten-free pasta, cooked al dente
1 cup or 2 small onions, cut into thin quarter-moons
1 cup or 2 carrots, halved lengthwise and cut into thin slices
2 cups or 1 package champignons/white button mushrooms or portobello mushrooms, wiped with a damp cloth and cut into 2 or 4 pieces each (cut the large ones into 4 and small ones into 2 pieces)
1 small bunch asparagus, cut into 2-inch pieces
1 tbsp garlic, minced
½ tbsp salt, or to taste
¾ tsp mixed Italian herbs (or ½ tsp sweet basil and a dash of sage, thyme and oregano)
¾ cups organic coconut cream
2–3 tbsp tahini
A few leaves of basil, for garnishing

Method:

1. Boil the pasta as per package instructions. Let the pasta be al dente (not overcooked). Overcooked pasta is not good for digestion.
2. Heat oil in a pan and add the onions and garlic with a pinch of sea salt. Sauté for 1–2 minutes. Add the mushrooms and cook for another 2–3 minutes.
3. Add the carrots and cook for 2–3 minutes. Add water as needed.
4. Add the asparagus and mix well. Stir in the coconut cream, tahini and herbs. Simmer for a few minutes.
5. Stir in the pasta just before serving. Adjust salt and seasoning to taste. Garnish and serve hot.

Tips and Variations:

1. If you need to re-heat the leftover pasta, then heat it on a low flame while adding a dash of water and stirring less to avoid breaking the pasta.

Quinoa Lemon Rice

Quinoa is high in iron, protein, calcium, magnesium and is an excellent addition to one's healing diet.

This recipe serves 3–4 people.

Ingredients:

1 cup quinoa, rinsed
1 large onion, chopped fine
12–14 curry leaves
1 dried red chilli
1 tbsp cumin seeds
1 tsp coriander, ground
1½–2 tsp ginger, minced
2 cloves of garlic, minced
2 tbsp fresh lemon juice
¼ tsp ground turmeric
2–2½ tsp sea salt, or to taste
2 tbsp organic or high-quality cold-pressed olive oil
¼ cup fresh coriander/cilantro

Method:

1. Add the quinoa and two cups of water, with a pinch of sea salt, into a stainless steel pot. After the first boil, lower the flame, place a flame tamer under the pot and simmer for 15–18 minutes or until the water dries up.

2. Turn off the flame, remove the cover and let it cool for at least half an hour. Stir with a bamboo spoon and move in a circular motion to ensure it stays fluffy.

3. Place a deep stainless steel or ceramic skillet on a medium–low flame. Add 2 tbsp olive oil and let it heat for 10–15 seconds. Add the cumin seeds, dried red chilli and the onion with ¼ tsp salt. Stir for 1–2 minutes. Add the turmeric, ground coriander, ginger, garlic, salt and broken curry leaves. Stir well.

4. Slowly add the cooked quinoa. Lower the flame and stir well for about a minute.

5. Turn off the flame and add the lemon juice and fresh coriander/cilantro leaves.

Tips and Variations:

1. Cook just before serving. If for some reason you are cooking it a while before serving, then don't add the lemon juice or coriander/cilantro leaves. Add these just before serving.

2. You may add chopped vegetables of your choice as well. Chop the vegetables small for better flavour.

3. You can also use red rice poha to add variation. All you need to do is soak the poha for 5–10 minutes and follow the same directions mentioned above. Remember that flattened rice flakes don't need to be cooked for 15–20 minutes like quinoa. You can add sweet peas and roasted unsalted peanuts to the dish.

4. You can also use barnyard millets, which are soft and mushy compared to quinoa. You can make an upma-style dish using the same seasoning as above. Of course you can use vegetables and seasonings of your choice.

17

Strengthening Protein Dishes

The body uses protein to build and repair. Proteins build the structure of our body, the bones, muscles, organs, skin, hair and blood. They also help in the communication, transmutation and transportation between the different body systems. With the right amount of protein, all bodily functions run smoothly and are maintained well.

Quantity of Protein

Unlike fat, the body does not store excess protein. The protein we eat is used as a source of energy to build and maintain the body. If we consume the right amount and quality of protein, our immune function gets a boost. If we consume very little protein, our body goes into a state of deprivation (since there is no stored protein as backup).

Protein deficiency affects focus, memory, circulation, heart health, metabolism, digestion and virtually every other function of the body. It also leads to the muscles shrinking, water retention, weakening of the nervous system and brain function, and memory loss. It is safe to say that if we don't consume the right amount of protein every day, the body will start deteriorating and collapsing.

On the other hand, too much protein is stored as fat, weakens the liver and increases the amount of uric acid in the blood, thereby damaging the kidneys. With a weak liver and kidneys, the amount of protein the body can handle also reduces, making the situation worse. Just like quicksand, everything sinks so quickly that we barely have the time, energy, structure or support to recover.

Quality of Protein

Ancient wisdom, and now ample research, says that a diet that has enough plant-based protein is beneficial. If consuming animal proteins, limit the quantity and improve the quality.

Plant-based proteins, which are rich in phytonutrients, like beans, lentils and bean products are high in fibre, stabilize hormones and blood sugar, lower cholesterol, aid heart health, improve lung and kidney health, and are low in saturated fats and high in minerals. For centuries, lentils and beans have been a daily staple in Indian diet. They have a protective effect on the immune function and general health. Beans, which resemble our kidneys, nourish them and the adrenal glands. Not only do they add to a person's strength, but they also help a person stay calm. When the kidneys are nourished, the excess energy in the lungs moves down towards them. If the kidneys are not functioning well, then the excess energy in the lungs accumulates and stagnates.

Usually, a smart plant-based protein is enough. However, if a person is switching from a diet rich in animal protein to a vegetarian diet, then a transition period may be required. Fish or other natural forms of animal protein are consumed in some parts of the world on a weekly or bi-weekly basis during the transition period.

People whose nervous systems and brains are used to a certain level of fat may never choose to transition to a smart plant-based diet. That, however, is a personal choice: whether one wishes to be vegetarian or have small quantities of high-quality animal protein. If one chooses to consume fish or poultry in small quantities, it is best to have the best-quality produce that is free of growth hormones, antibiotics, contamination and environmental toxins.

Here are some recipes you can try:

1. Mixed Healing Lentils (page 154)
2. Red Lobia/ Kulath ki Dal (page 156)
3. Green Moong Dal (page 158)
4. Vegetable Sambar (page 159)
5. Besan Chila with Leeks (page 161)
6. Kala Chana Tikkis (page 162)
7. Yellow Moong Dal (page 164)
8. Basil Hummus (page 165)
9. Red Lobia Burgers (page 166)
10. Coconut Fish Stew (page 167)
11. Fish in Mustard-Carom Seed Marinade (page 167)
12. Gingery Fish Stew (page 168)
13. Mixed Bean Salad(page 169)

Mixed Healing Lentils

Horse gram lentil (kulath ki dal) is known to clear kidney stones. They are also beneficial for people with asthma, bronchitis, urinary tract infections and diabetes. Together with split chickpeas (chana dal) and red lentils (masoor dhuli), they make for a nourishing creamy dish. I highly recommend weekly use of this lentil.

The recipe below makes 4–6 servings.

Ingredients:

½ cup horse gram lentil, rinsed and soaked overnight in three cups of water
½ cup red lentils, rinsed 4–6 times until the water is clear
½ cup split chickpeas, rinsed 3–4 times
1½ cups of pumpkin, cut into small cubes
1 tsp cumin seeds
¼ tsp ground turmeric
1 de-seeded green chilli, diced small
2 tbsp ginger, minced
1 tbsp garlic, minced or crushed
1 tbsp lemon juice, or to taste
¾–1 tbsp powdered jaggery or any other natural sweetener (not honey as it should not be boiled)
A pinch of black pepper
2 tbsp cold-pressed organic sesame oil

Method:

1. Put the horse gram lentil and the soaking water into a large pressure cooker. After the first whistle, lower the flame and simmer for 30–35 minutes. Turn off the flame and let it cool down.
2. Open the pressure cooker and add the other two lentils along with turmeric and two cups of water. Bring to one whistle and let it simmer for 5–10 minutes. Turn off the flame and let it cool.

3. In a separate deep stainless steel skillet, heat the oil and add the cumin seeds, ginger, garlic and green chilies. Sauté for 1–2 minutes and then add the pumpkin. Sauté for another 1–2 minutes. Add the lentils to this pot along with a cup of warm water. Bring to a boil and then lower the flame. Add the salt and powdered jaggery and simmer for 5–10 minutes. Do not overcook else the flavour of the ginger and garlic will fade. Stir in the lemon juice and black pepper and adjust the seasoning to taste. Serve hot.

Tips and Variations:

1. If horse gram lentil is not available where you live, you may use red black-eyed beans (red lobia) or aduki beans.
2. You can also try making kasuri methi (fenugreek leaves, which are rich in minerals) and split chickpea lentil. This dish uses a little more oil.

Red Lobia/Kulath ki Dal

Softly cooked red lobia is excellent sssfor fighting infections and supporting the immune function. They are good for the kidneys too.

This recipe serves 4 people.

Ingredients:

1 cup red lobia, or runner beans/pinto beans soaked in 3 cups water overnight
1 large onion, cut into quarter-moons
1½ cup carrots, cut into small cubes

1½ cups pumpkin, cut into small cubes
1 tbsp powdered jaggery or any other natural sweetener
1–1½ tbsp cold-pressed organic sesame oil
1½ tsp organic ghee (optional)
1 tbsp whole cumin seeds
1 tbsp ginger
½ tsp ground turmeric
1 green chilli, cut small
1 tsp sea salt, or to taste
2–3 tbsp fresh coriander leaves/cilantro or flat-leaf parsley

Method:

1 Put the soaked beans along with the water into a pressure cooker. Cook on a medium–high flame. Let it come to a pressure, or wait for 2–3 whistles, and then lower the flame. Place a flame tamer under the pressure cooker and cook for 45 minutes. Turn off the flame and let it cool. Do not place under cold running water.

2 In a deep stainless steel skillet, heat the oil and sauté the cumin seeds for 30 seconds. Add the onions, ginger and green chillies with a pinch of salt. Sauté for another 2–3 minutes. Add the pumpkin and turmeric with a dash of water and cook for another 5 minutes, covered on a simmer flame. Add the carrots and ground cumin and cook for another 2–3 minutes.

3 Add the powdered jaggery and some water from the cooked beans and simmer for 3–4 minutes. Add the beans to the vegetables and mix well. Add salt to taste. Cook for another 5 minutes and add 1½ tsps of organic ghee. Serve hot with brown rice or unyeasted sourdough bread, chapatti or corn tortillas.

Tips and Variations:

1. You can use pinto beans, kidney beans, aduki beans or runner beans in this recipe.
2. You can use ¼ cup beans instead of 1 cup and make it a soup. The dark water from the red lobia is known to be rich in minerals and good for the kidneys. If someone has dark circles around their eyes, this dish is particularly good for them.
3. You can also add a little bit of barley or brown rice and make it a soupy khichdi.
4. You can add 1–2 tsps organic ghee for better digestion or for an added flavour for fussy eaters who want rich food during the transition period.

Green Moong Dal

Moong beans are considered one of the healthiest according to Ayurveda. They are considered to be *tridoshic*, which means that it balances all the three doshas—vata, kapha and pitta.

Ingredients:

¾ cup whole or split green moong dal, rinsed and soaked in 3 cups of drinking water for 2–4 hours
½ cup carrots, minced or cut into small cubes
1 large or 2 small dried red chillies
2 tsp cumin seeds
1 tsp ground coriander
4–5 cloves of garlic, pressed or minced
1 tbsp cold-pressed sesame oil or organic ghee
A pinch of ground turmeric

1 tsp sea salt, or to taste
2–3 tbsp fresh cilantro or parsley, for garnishing

Method:

1. Bring the green moong dal along with the water and another 2 cups of water to a boil or pressure in a stainless steel pan. Lower the flame, place a flame tamer at the bottom and cook for 45 minutes. Turn off the flame and let it cool naturally.
2. In a separate stainless skillet, add the ghee along with the dried red chillies, cumin seeds, ground coriander, ground turmeric and garlic. Lower the flame and stir for about ½–1 minute until the garlic is fragrant and turns light brown. Add the salt and stir well. Turn off the flame and transfer this to the pot with cooked lentils. Adjust salt to taste. Add ½–1 cup water if the lentils are too thick and simmer for about a minute.
3. Garnish with fresh cilantro and serve hot.

Vegetable Sambar

This is a south Indian spicy and sour lentil dish that is usually served with fermented steamed rice cakes, rice or fermented savoury pancakes.

Ingredients:

¾ cup split pigeon peas (toor dal, tuvar dal), rinsed 4–5 times
1 drumstick, cut into 2-inch pieces
¼ cup or 1 small onion, cut into quarter-moons
¼ cup green beans

½ cup pumpkin or ash gourd, cut into small cubes
¼ cup carrots, cut into small cubes or thin diagonal half-moons
¼ cup okra, cut into ½–1 inch pieces
10–12 curry leaves
½ tsp small reddish brown or black mustard seeds
¼ tsp cumin seeds
1 heaping tbsp de-seeded tamarind, soaked in ¼ cup water for 30 minutes
1 tomato, de-seeded and cut small
2 cloves of garlic, minced
1 tsp ginger, minced (optional)
A generous pinch of hing
¼ tsp ground turmeric
1½ tsp powdered jaggery
1 large or 2 small dried red chillies (optional, do not use if condition is aggravated)
1½ tsp sea salt or to taste (should be just enough to bring out the flavours)
1 tbsp organic cold-pressed coconut oil or organic ghee
1–1½ tsp sambar masala

Method:

1. Bring the lentils and 4½ cups of water to a boil in a stainless steel pot. Lower the flame to the lowest and place a flame tamer under the pot. Cook covered for 35–40 minutes.
2. Place a stainless steel skillet on a medium flame and heat 1 tbsp coconut oil or ghee. Add the mustard seeds, cumin seeds and dried red chilies. When the mustard seeds begin to splutter, add the ginger, garlic, onion and ¼ tsp salt. Stir for 30–60 seconds. Add the tomatoes and lower the flame, and cook covered for about 2 minutes. Add ¼ cup water and cook for another 2–3 minutes.

3. Squeeze or blend the tamarind (without any seeds) and strain to save the sour liquid.
4. After the lentils are cooked, remove the flame tamer and bring to a boil. Add the pumpkin and drumsticks and cook on medium heat for about 5–7 minutes. Add the carrots and cook for another minute. Add the green beans and okra and cook for another minute.
5. Add the tomato–onion–garlic mix to the lentils and mix well.
6. Season the lentils with the sambar masala and powdered jaggery, sour tamarind liquid and hing. Adjust salt and seasonings to taste. Serve hot with idlis (steamed rice cake/bread), rice or appams (steamed rice pancakes).

Tips and Variations:

1. Be careful to ensure that the oil does not smoke while waiting for the seeds to splutter. If that happens, turn off the flame, wipe and wash the pot and start again. Smoked oil is dangerous for health.

Besan Chila with Leeks (Savoury Spiced Gram Flour Pancakes)

This recipe makes 3–4 six-inch wide pancakes.

Ingredients:

1 cup gram flour
¾–1 cup water (more water will make a thinner and lighter chila)
½ tsp sea salt, or to taste
½ tsp ground cumin
¼ tsp ground turmeric

½–1 tsp or 1–2 small green chillies, minced
1 tsp ginger, minced
⅓ cup leeks, cut lengthwise into half and then into thin slices
About ½ tsp organic cold-pressed sesame oil or organic ghee per pancake

Method:

1. Mix the gram flour and water. Add the vegetables and seasoning. Mix well to ensure there are no lumps.
2. Heat the oil in a ceramic coated pan. Pour ¼ the batter with a large ladle and spread thin into a circle like a pancake. Lower the flame and cook covered for 1–2 minutes. Once you see a bubble forming on the top of the pancake, and it looks almost cooked, carefully flip it upside down and cook for 1–2 minutes. Remove the pan away from the heat and with a half-cut onion or a clean paper towel wipe out the old oil.
3. Serve hot.

Tips and Variations:

1. Before making the pancakes, make a test pancake to check the seasoning.

Kala Chana Tikkis

Dark brown chickpeas (kala chana) are often served in temples in India, as it revered as a food for immortality. It is rich in minerals and excellent for the spleen–kidney channel. It also improves heart, lung and hormonal health.

Ingredients:

1 cup dark brown chickpeas, soaked overnight and boiled or pressure-cooked until soft
1–1½ tsp garlic, minced
3–4 tsps mango powder (amchur)
2 tsp ground cumin
1¼ tsp–1½ tsp garam masala to taste (keep it slightly stronger than you would like as the aroma and flavour reduces a little after frying)
1–1½ tsp or 2–3 green chillies, de-seeded and cut (sometimes 1½ chillies are enough and sometimes more may be required)
1–1½ tsp sea salt, or to taste
1 tsp ground coriander

Method:

1. Mash the chickpeas, with just a little water, to a smooth consistency. The consistency should be like that of peanut butter or hummus.
2. Place the mashed chickpeas in a bowl and add the seasonings. The seasoning should be slightly on the stronger side as the taste will reduce once fried. Make 1¼-inch balls and press from the top and bottom.
3. Pan-fry or deep fry and serve with cilantro–mint or cilantro–mango chutney.

Tips and Variations:

1. You may use bread crumbs or gram flour (besan) to make the patties crunchier.

Yellow Moong Dal

This recipe serves 3–4 people.

Ingredients:

1 cup yellow moong lentil, rinsed 3–4 times
4–5 cups water, add water as desired
½ tsp sea salt, or to taste
¼ tsp ground turmeric
1 tsp ginger, minced
1 tbsp organic ghee (optional)
1–2 tbsp fresh coriander/cilantro leaves, or fresh spring onion/ scallions

Method:

1. Bring the lentil, water and a pinch of salt, ginger, turmeric to a boil. Lower the flame and simmer for 30–35 minutes.
2. Adjust salt to taste and add the ghee.
3. Garnish and serve hot.

Tips and Variations:

1. You may heat any organic oil or ghee in a pan and fry 1–2 tsp cumin seeds and 1 de-seeded green chilli for added flavour.
2. You can also use half-yellow moong and half-red lentils in the recipe.

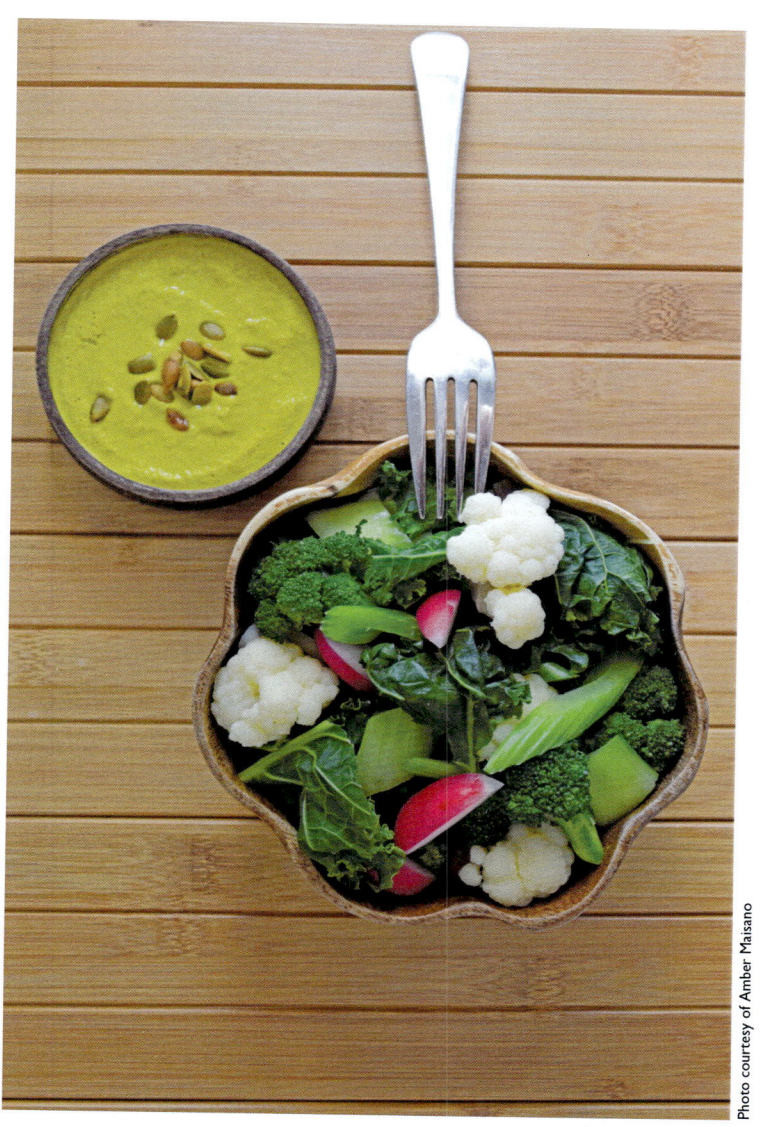

Kale and Vegetable Salad with Carrot Dressing (see page 259)

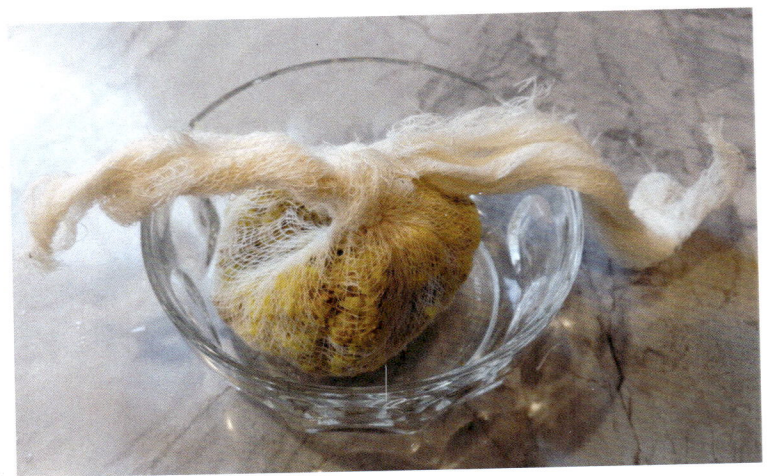

Ginger Compress (see page 74)

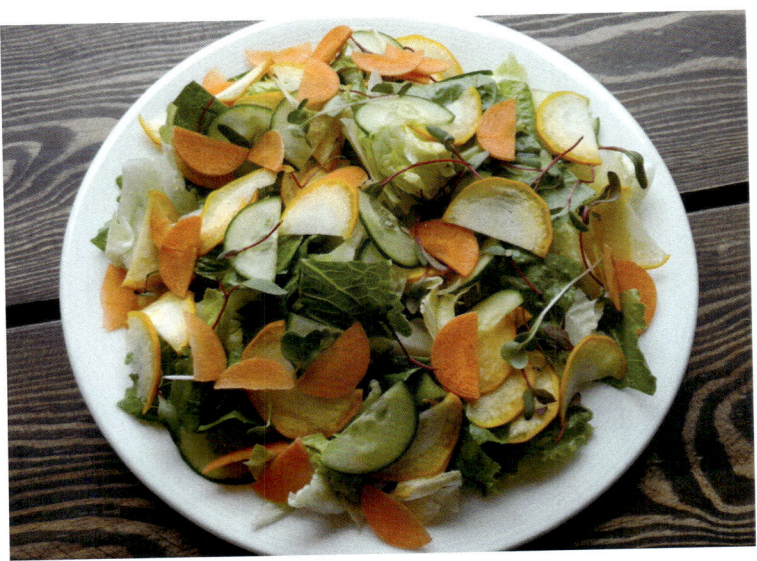

Zucchini, Cucumber and Microgreens Salad (see page 188)

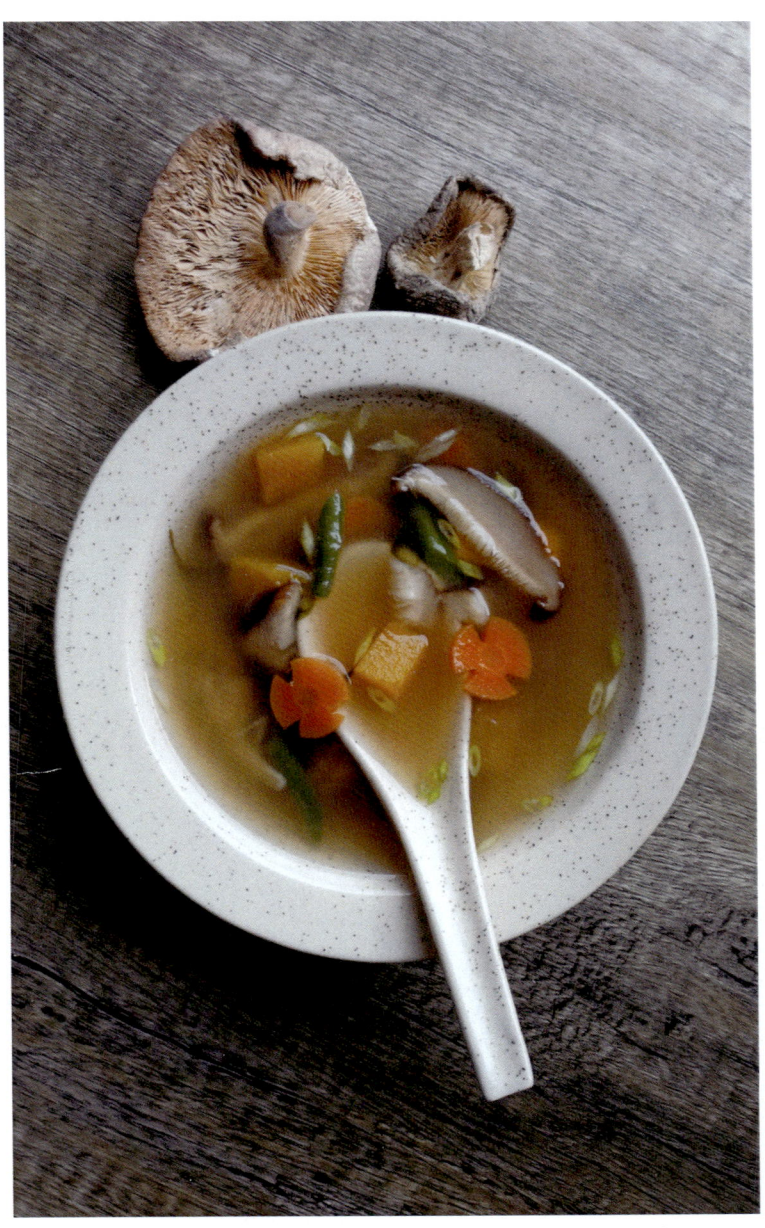

Miso Soup with White Radish (see page 243)

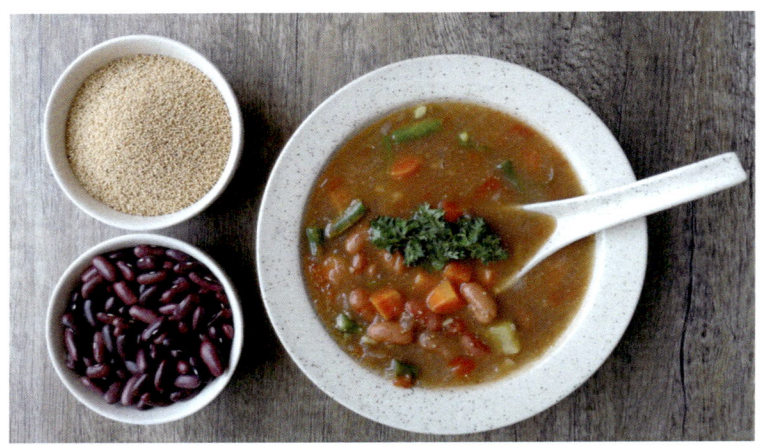

Amaranth and Kidney Bean Soup (see page 126)

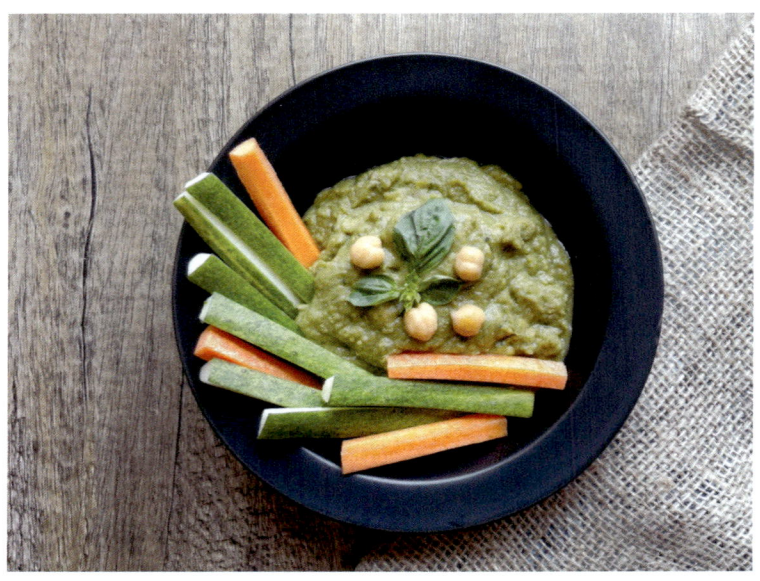

Basil Hummus (see page 165)

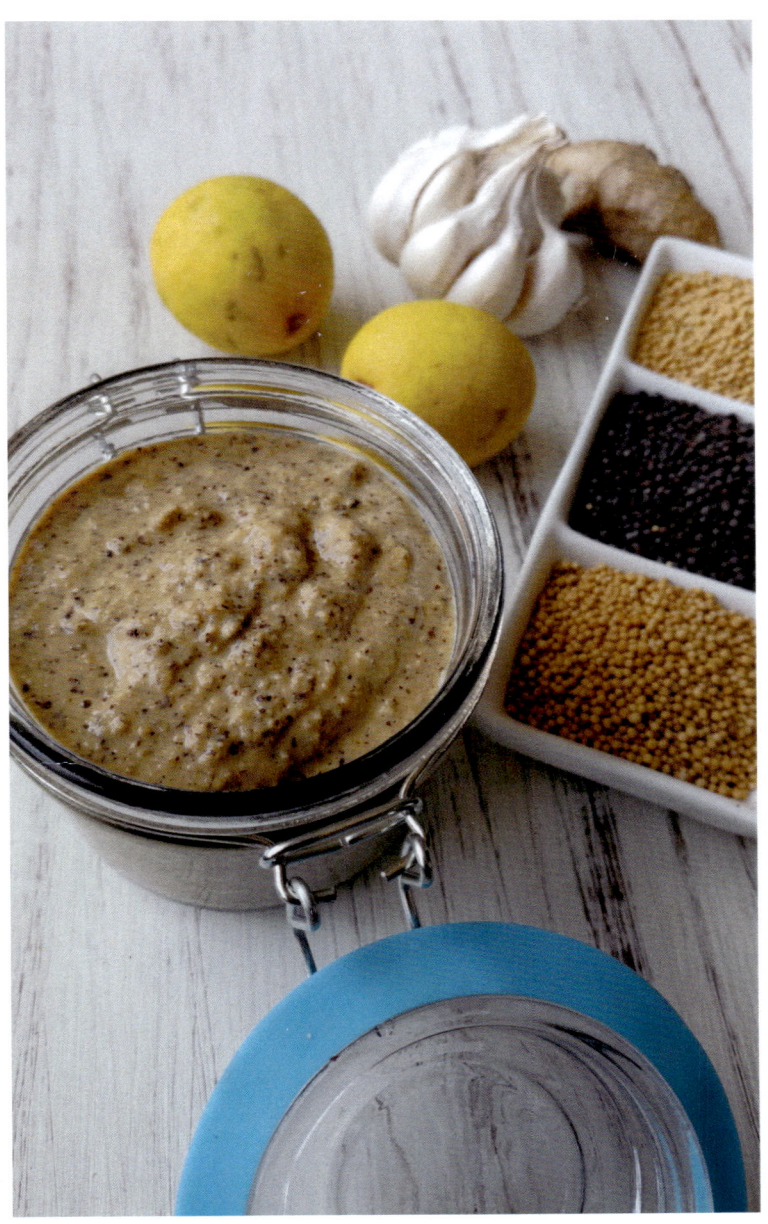

Home-made Mustard Spread (see page 202)

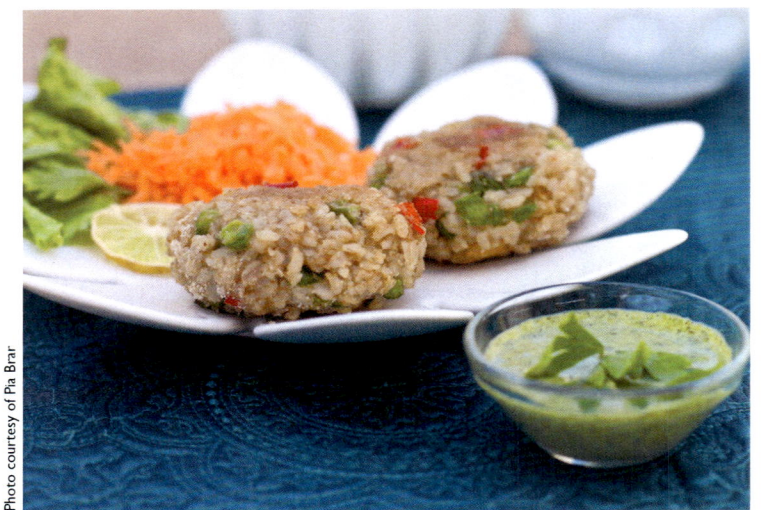

Mona's Brown Rice Tikkis (see page 144)

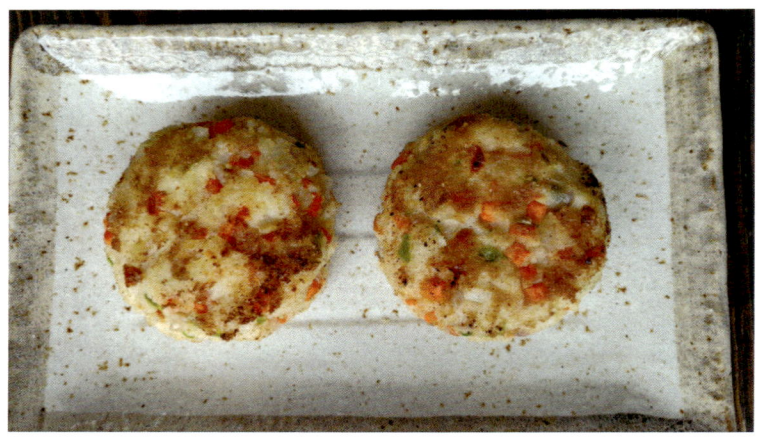

Millet and Vegetable Tikkis (see page 139)

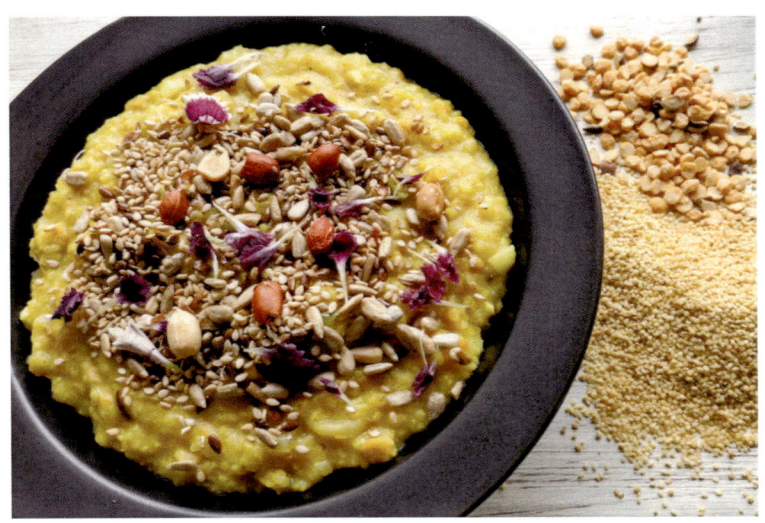

Black Millet and Chana Dal Khichdi (see page 138)

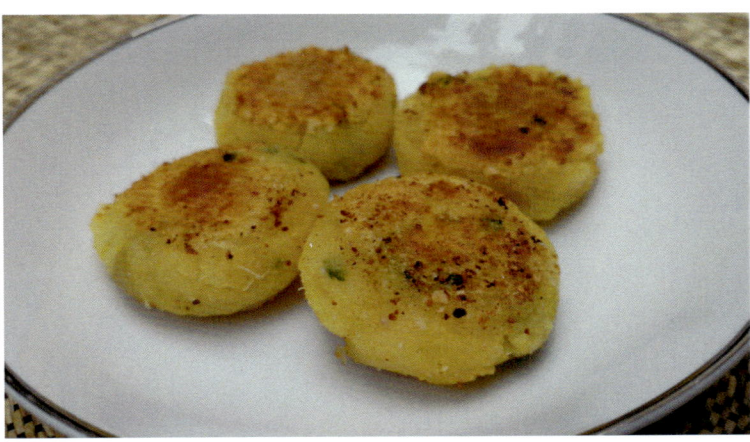

Sweet Potato Tikkis (see page 178)

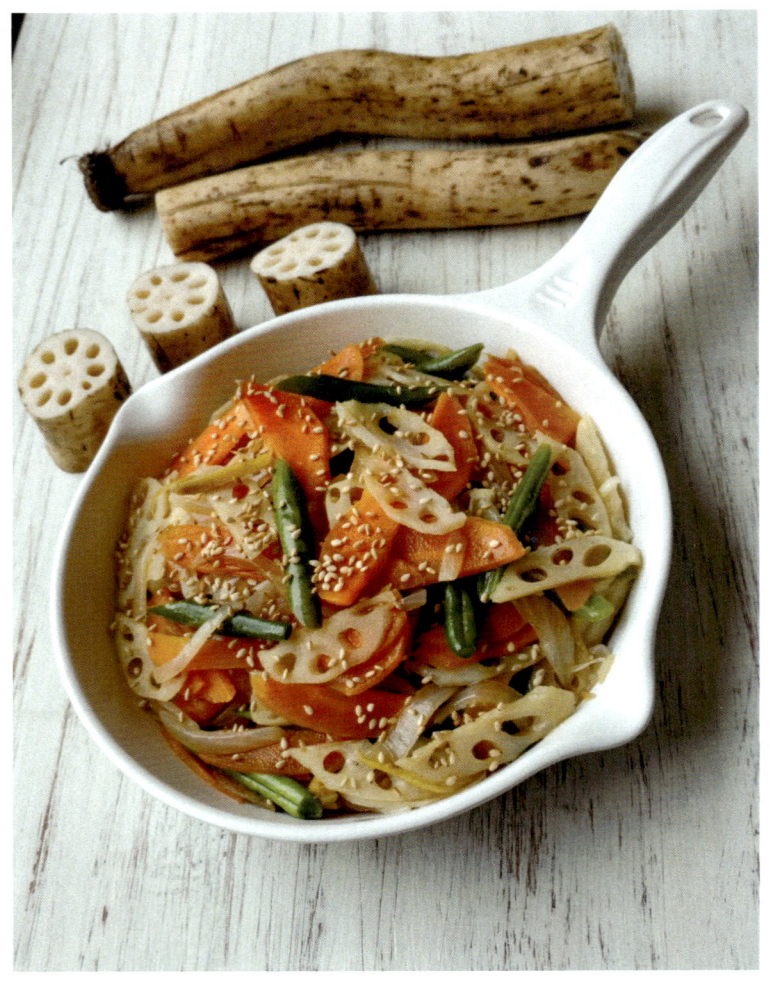

Lotus and Vegetable Stir-fry (see page 179)

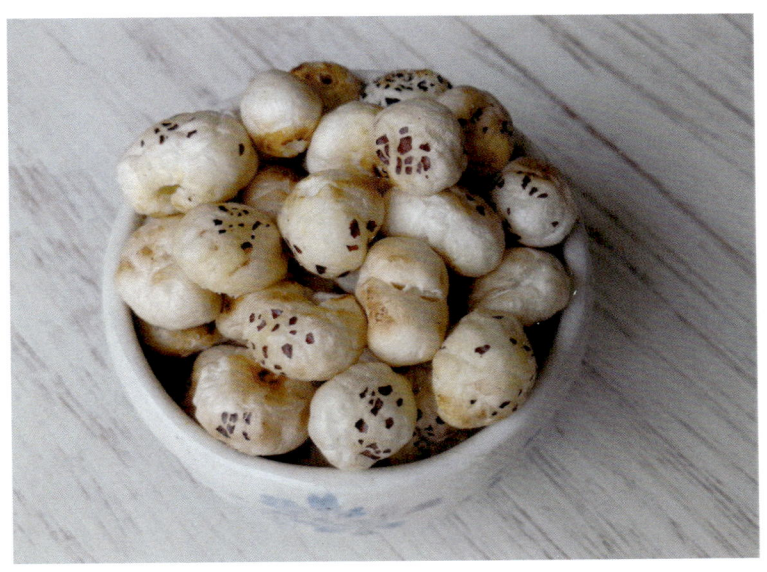

Roasted Lotus Seed Makhane (see page 216)

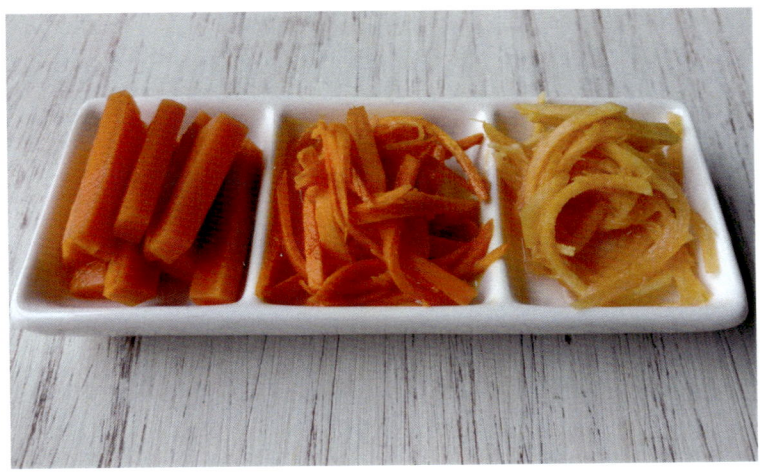

Oil-free Carrot, Turmeric and Ginger Pickles (see page 194)

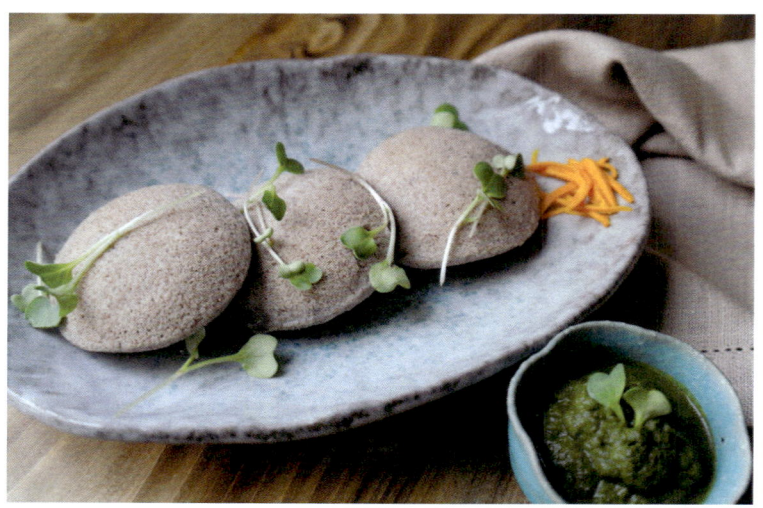

Wholegrain Idlis (see pages 145 and 147)

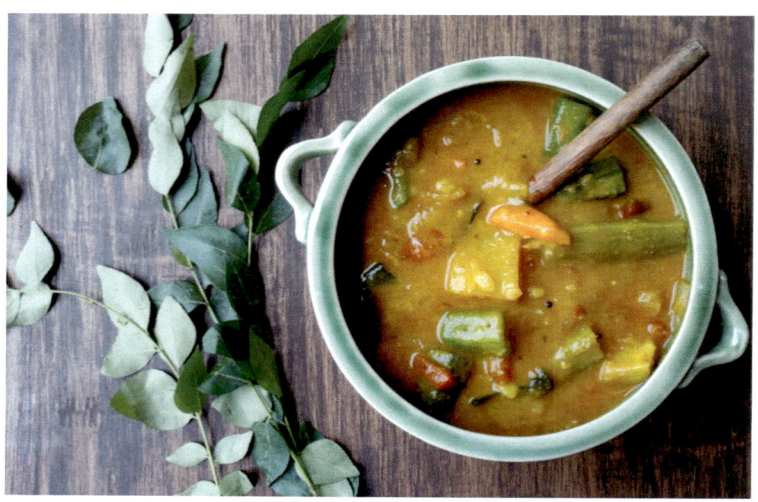

Vegetable Sambar (see page 159)

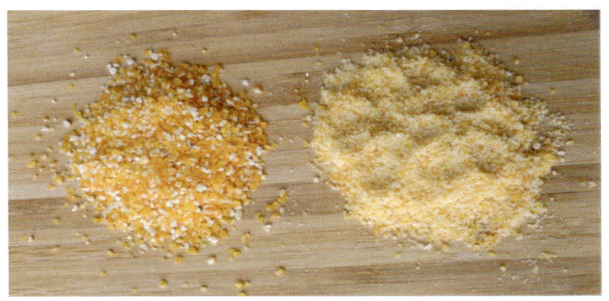

Corn dalia before and after being ground

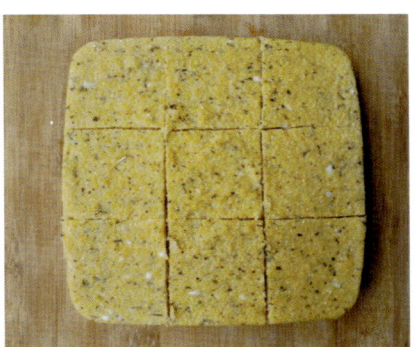

Polenta Squares

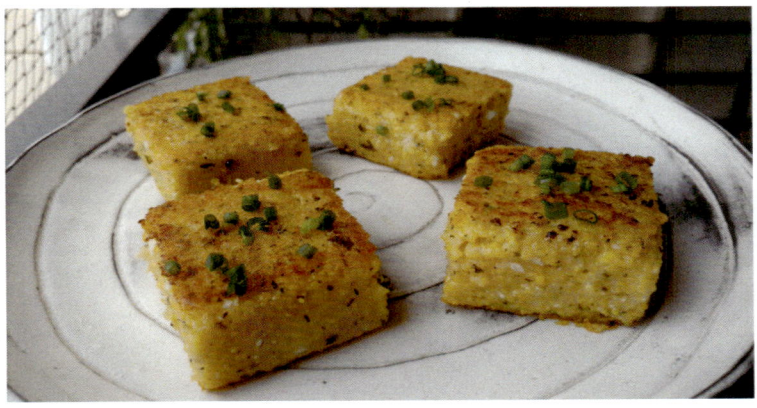

Pan-fried Polenta Squares (see page 141)

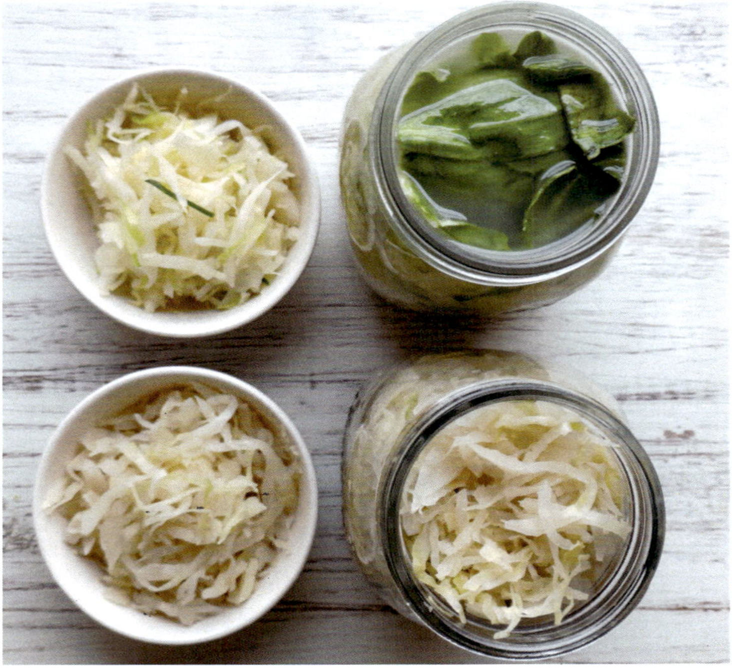

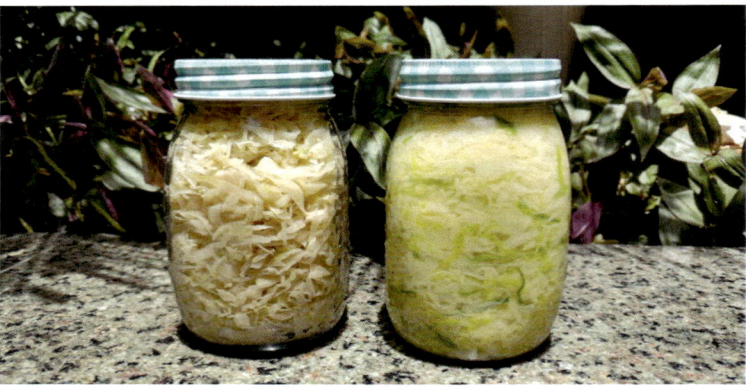

Pickling sauerkraut in a jar (top right) requires a cabbage leaf. Use the leaf to cover the vegetables and press it down to ensure that the pickling liquid completely covers the vegetables and the leaf (see page 193)

Pickled sauerkraut on the first day (right), on the tenth day (left)

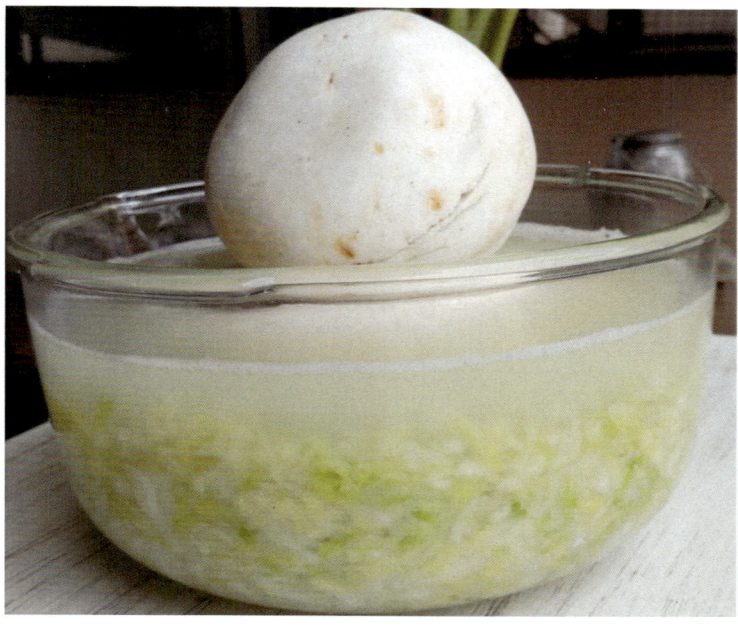

If you are making a large quantity of sauerkraut, use a ceramic or glass pickling pot and place a ceramic plate on it. You can then place a heavy stone and press it down so that the liquid covers the plate

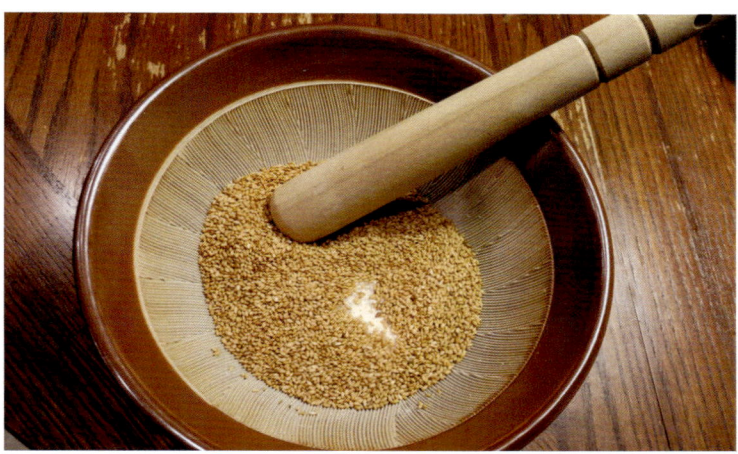

Home-made sesame seed salt in a mortar and pestle (see page 196)

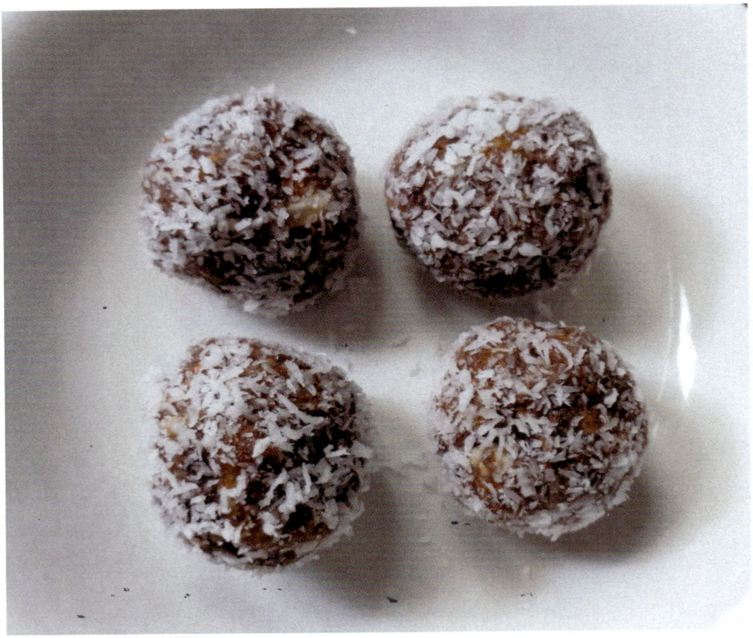

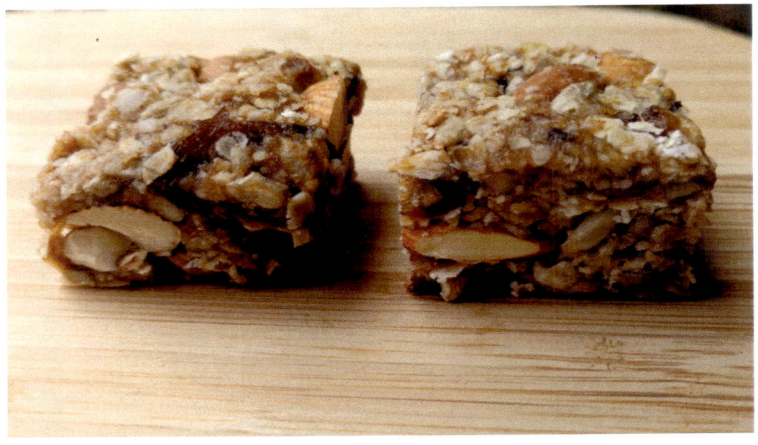

Date–Fig Balls (see page 218)

Granola Squares (see page 217)

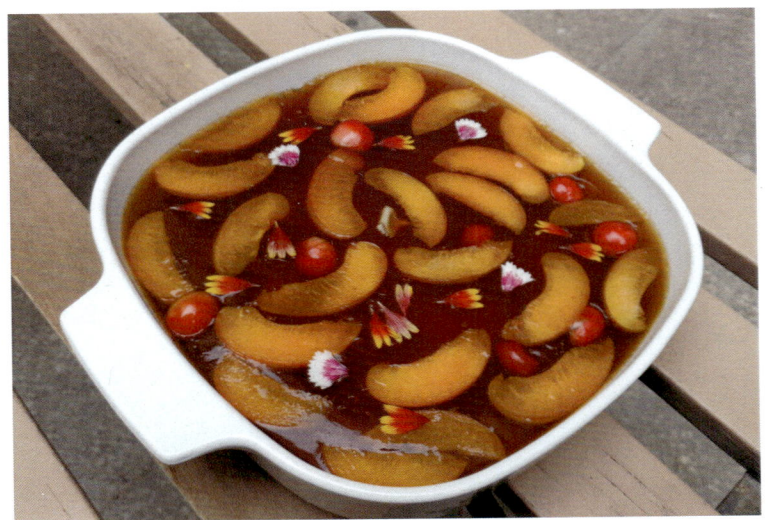

Apricot Kanten (see page 213)

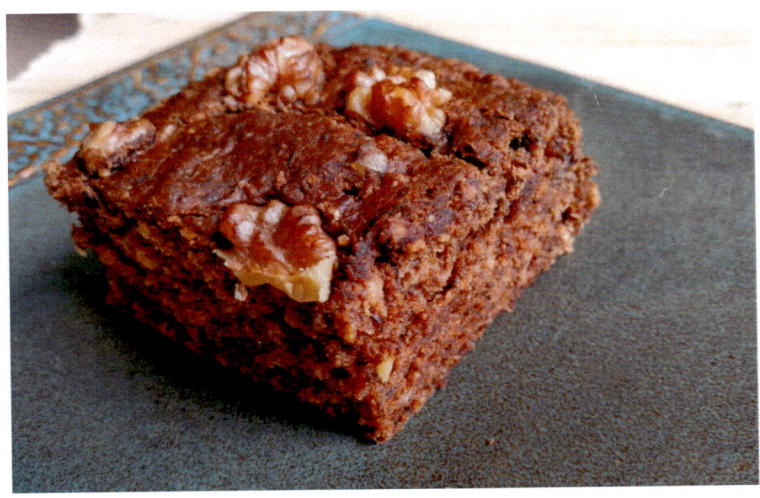

Vegan Banana Bread (see page 223)

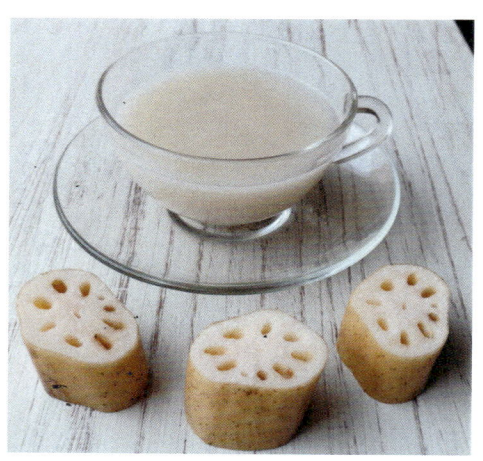

Lotus Root Tea (see page 72)

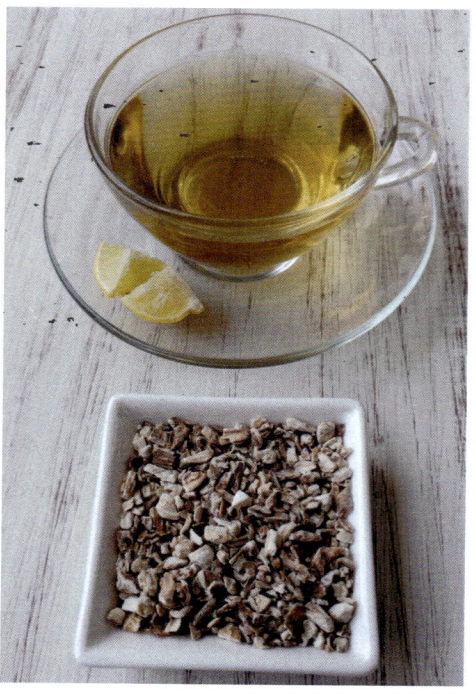

Burdock Tea (see page 73)

Basil Hummus

This is a yummy and easy-to-digest way of having beans. Basil is known to have anti-inflammatory, anti-bacterial and anti-aging properties.

This recipe serves 3–4 people.

Ingredients:

1 cup chickpeas, rinsed and soaked in 3 cups water overnight
1 tbsp or 1–2 cloves of garlic, freshly crushed
2½–3 packed cups fresh organic Italian basil, hard stems and bad leaves removed
5–6 fresh tulsi leaves
3½–4 tbsp lemon juice, or to taste
¾ tsp sea salt, or to taste
1–2 green chillies, de-seeded and cut small
2 tbsp tahini

Method:

1. Discard the soaking water and boil or pressure-cook until the beans are soft. Let it cool.
2. Blend all the ingredients to a smooth and thick consistency. Do not add all the water from cooking the beans. Add a little at first and add more if needed. You can refrigerate this for up to 2–3 days.

Tips and Variations:

1. You may use roasted garlic instead of raw garlic. Roast garlic with a drizzle of olive oil and a dash of salt in

the oven at 220°C. If using a whole pod, cut off the top and drizzle oil and a dash of salt and roast for about 25 minutes. If roasting peeled cloves, roast for 10–15 minutes. Watch closely. You can make extra and store it in the refrigerator for up to 7–10 days.

Red Lobia Burgers

Creating a variety in textures and flavours is an essential part of cooking for wellness. This is a hearty and delicious bean burger recipe that is often liked by both children and adults.

This recipe serves 4–5 people.

Ingredients:

1 cup red lobia, rinsed and soaked overnight
1 cup carrots, cut very small (almost minced)
½ cup celery
1 medium onion, minced
1½ tsp ground cumin
A tiny pinch of ground turmeric
1 tsp ground thyme
2–3 cloves of garlic, minced
Breadcrumbs from unyeasted sourdough bread or gram flour
Cold-pressed organic sesame oil for pan-frying

Method:

1. Pressure-cook or boil the beans until soft.
2. Pan-fry the vegetables and season to taste.

3. Mix and make burgers (follow recipe like millet vegetable croquettes on page 139 but use mashed beans instead of millets).
4. Dust with besan or bread crumbs and pan-fry until light brown.

Coconut Fish Stew

This is a mildly sweet and creamy fish preparation. You can serve it with steamed idlis, appams or rice. It is a variation of the coconut vegetable stew on page 181.

Lightly marinate the fish using a little lemon and garlic. Add the stew towards the end and cook for 3–4 minutes till the fish is well cooked.

Fish in Mustard–Carom Seed Marinade

This is a traditional Indian recipe that uses a freshly prepared mustard and carom marinade. Mustard helps cut through mucus and toxic buildup in the lungs.

This recipe serves 3–4 people.

Ingredients:

Boneless surmai or sole, 400 gms, cut like small fish tikkas
2–3 tbsp mustard oil for pan-frying

Mustard Marinade

½ cup for marination
2–3 tbsp for adding in the end

Method:

1. Marinade the fish in 2 tbsp lemon juice and ¾ cup home-made mustard marinade for two hours. The marinade should just about cover the fish. Don't use all of the marinade.
2. Pan-fry the fish on a low flame for 2–3 minutes or until the fish is well-cooked on both sides. Remove from heat and transfer this into a glass or ceramic serving bowl. Mix 2–3 tbsp of raw mustard marinade into the cooked fish to taste (use less as the mustard marinade has a sharp taste).
3. Serve hot.

Tips and Variations:

1. Use less marinade at the end. Serve alongside at the table for those who want a stronger flavour.

Gingery Fish Stew

This recipe serves 4 people.

Ingredients:

500 gm boneless surmai, singhara or sole
2/3 cup or 160 ml organic, or freshly pressed coconut milk
2 onions, diced
1 tomato de-seeded, diced
4 tbsp ginger, minced
2–3 tbsp garlic, crushed or pressed
3–4 tbsp cold-pressed coconut oil
2–3 green chillies, de-seeded and diced
½ tsp ground cinnamon

¼–½ tsp ground cardamom to taste
½ tsp black pepper, freshly ground
½ tsp turmeric
2 tsp sea salt, or to taste

Method:

1. Wash and marinate the fish in ¼ tsp turmeric, 2 tsp crushed garlic and 1 tbsp lemon juice for 2 hours.
2. Puree the onions to a smooth paste with ¼ cup water.
3. Heat 2 tbsp of coconut oil in a stainless steel skillet and add the onions with ½ tsp sea salt. Sauté for 1–2 minutes and then lower the flame and cook covered for 7–10 minutes.
4. Puree the tomato, ginger, garlic and green chilies with 1/3 cup of water.
5. Add this to the onions along with 1 tsp sea salt and sauté. Continue to cook on a low flame for another 12–15 minutes.
6. Add the coconut milk and 1–1½ cups water to desired consistency and stir well. Add only enough water as you would like the consistency of the curry to be. Adjust salt to taste and simmer for another 3–5 minutes. Add the pepper and simmer for another 2 minutes. Serve hot with rice, appams or chapattis.
7. In a separate ceramic or stainless steel flat pan, pan-fry the fish on both sides in 1–2 tbsp coconut oil on a medium low flame for 2–3 minutes, or until the fish is done. Mix the fish into the gingery spicy coconut curry just before serving.

Mixed Bean Salad

This recipe serves 4 people.

Ingredients:

½ cup white chickpeas (garbanzo beans), rinsed and soaked overnight and pressured-cooked until soft

½ cup black chickpeas, rinsed and soaked overnight and pressure-cooked or boiled until soft

2 tbsp sprouted moong beans, steamed for 2 minutes

½ fresh cilantro, cut small

1 small or ½ cup onions, cut very small

¼ tsp sea salt, or to taste

2 tbsp lemon juice, or to taste

Method:

1. Let the beans cool to room temperature. Mix all the ingredients and serve at room temperature.

18

Cleansing Vegetable Dishes

Natural systems of medicine that are energy-based have a clear understanding about how the food we eat travels to different parts of the body. Foods that resemble a certain part of the body usually nourish those organ systems.

As far as asthma and lung-related diseases are concerned, it is absolutely critical to bring attention to these questions:

1. Which vegetables are mucus-forming and which are mucus-dissolving?
2. Which vegetables are inflammatory and which are anti-inflammatory?
3. Which vegetables specifically strengthen the lungs and immune function?
4. Which foods improve blood quality, so that the body is less prone to allergies, infections and reactions?

You can turn to page 67 to refer to the list of healthy and harmful vegetables. Listed below are some recipes you can try.

1. Pumpkin Subzi (Kaddu) (page 172)

Pumpkin Subzi

Pumpkin is good for the digestion and immune system. It is naturally sweet and hence promotes healthy blood sugar levels too. Pumpkin also gives stability to the hormonal and nervous systems.

This recipe serves 2 people.

Ingredients:

2 cups pumpkin, cut into small cubes
1 large or 2 small dried red chillies, wiped to remove any dust, broken into half
1½ tsps cumin seeds
2–2½ tsp sea salt, or to taste
1½ tbsp organic cold-pressed sesame oil
2½ tsp ginger, minced
¼ tsp ground turmeric

1 tsp mango powder (amchur)
1½–2 tbsp powdered jaggery, or to taste
½ tsp fenugreek seeds

Method:

1. In a deep stainless steel skillet, heat the oil and add the dried red chilies, cumin, fenugreek seeds and ginger. Sauté for 30–40 seconds and then add the pumpkin, salt and turmeric. Stir well and cook for another ½–1 minute.
2. Add ¾–1 cup water and bring to a slight boil. Lower the flame and let simmer. Cook covered for 10–12 minutes, until the pumpkin is cooked and the water has almost dried. Add the powdered jaggery and mango powder and adjust the salt to taste. Turn off the flame and let it cook a little bit before roughly mashing it with a masher. Serve warm–hot.

Bottle Gourd Subzi

This recipe serves 2–3 people.

Ingredients:

4 cups or 2 small bottle gourds, cut into small cubes or thin half-moons (peel if not organic)
1/2 cup or 1 tomato, cut small, de-seeded
1 cup or 2 small onions, cut into small or into thin half-moons (match the cut to that of the gourd)
1 green chilli, de-seeded and cut
1 clove of garlic, minced (optional)
½ tsp black pepper

1 tbsp organic cold-pressed sesame oil, or high-quality cold-pressed olive oil, or organic ghee
2 tsp sea salt, or to taste

Method:

1. Heat oil in a deep stainless steel skillet. Add the onions and ½ tsp sea salt. Sauté for 20–30 seconds.
2. Add the garlic, green chillies and tomatoes and 1 tsp salt and sauté for another 2 minutes. Add a dash of water to avoid burning.
3. Stir in the bottle gourd and ⅓–½ cup water and mix well. Simmer for about 7–10 minutes. Add the remaining salt and pepper and adjust to taste. Serve hot.

White Radish and Greens Subzi

White radish is pungent and helps melt extra fat and mucus buildup. The greens are rich in minerals and cleanse the endocrine and immune systems.

This recipe serves 2–3 people.

Ingredients:

3 cups packed white radish, halved lengthwise and cut into thin half-moons
4 cups white radish leaves, finely chopped (keep stems separate)
1 tbsp and 1 tsp organic cold-pressed sesame oil
½ tsp cumin seeds
¼ tsp ground turmeric
1½ tbsp ginger, minced

1 tsp or 1–2 cloves of garlic, crushed or minced
1 tsp sea salt, or to taste

Method:

1. Heat oil in a stainless steel or Le Crueset deep wok or pan. Add the cumin seeds, ginger and garlic and sauté for 30–60 seconds. Stir in the white radish, salt and turmeric. Sauté for 1–2 minutes on a medium heat. Add a dash of water if needed.
2. Add the finely chopped stems and ¼ cup water and mix well. Sauté for 1–2 minutes.
3. Add the remaining leaves, stir well and lower the flame. Sauté for a few more minutes, or until it is cooked and the water has dried. Adjust salt to taste. Serve hot.

Tips and Variations:

1. You may add ½ tsp lemon juice.
2. You may add 1–2 de-seeded green chillies to taste.

Gingery Carrot and Peas Subzi

This is a traditional nourishing winter dish from north India.
This recipe serves 2–3 people.

Ingredients:

1½ cups of carrots, cut into small cubes (red carrots taste the best as they are naturally sweet)
1½ cup sweet peas
2 tbsp ginger, minced

½ tsp black pepper
1 tbsp organic cold-pressed sesame oil or organic ghee
1 tsp sea salt, or to taste
2 tbsp fresh coriander/cilantro for garnishing

Method:

1. Heat the oil or ghee in a stainless steel or ceramic skillet and add the ginger. Sauté on a low flame. Stir in the peas and sauté for another 2 minutes. Add a dash of water if needed.
2. Add the carrots. Mix well and sauté for another minute. Add ¼ cup of water and cook covered on a low flame for about 8–10 minutes or until soft. Add a dash of water if needed and adjust salt to taste. Add the black pepper and stir well. Garnish and serve hot.

Tips and Variations:

1. This dish tastes best with organic ghee.
2. You can also try south Indian-style green beans. Use two sprigs of curry leaves and ½ tsp mustard seed in the beginning with the cold-pressed organic coconut oil. Stir in 2–3 tbsp grated or dessicated coconut just before removing from the flame.

Stir-Fried Amaranth Greens

Amaranth greens, commonly called chaulai saag, is a blood purifier and is considered beneficial for the respiratory and digestive systems.

I recommend using it twice or thrice a week when in season. This recipe serves 2–3 people.

Ingredients:

5–6 packed cups amaranth greens, washed well to remove all dirt and roughly chopped (keep the stems separately)
½ cup carrots, cut into thin quarter-moons
1 cup or 1 medium onion, cut small (optional)
2–3 cloves of garlic, pressed or minced
¾ tbsp organic cold-pressed sesame oil or organic cold-pressed coconut oil
½ tsp sea salt, or to taste
½ cup sprouts of your choice
Lemon juice to taste

Method:

1. Heat oil in a stainless steel skillet and add the garlic. Sauté for 30 seconds on a medium flame. Add the onions and ¼ tsp sea salt and sauté for 1–2 minutes.
2. Add the stem first and the leaves 2 minutes later. Sauté for another 1–2 minutes. Add the sprouts and adjust salt to taste. Squeeze a dash of fresh lemon juice just before serving. Serve warm–hot.

Tips and Variations:

1. Amaranth greens shrink after cooking. Make more and keep this in mind while planning a meal.

Pan-Fried Lotus Root

When you cut a lotus root, the cross-section looks like the lungs with the bronchi. Lotus root grows under water and, when consumed, pulls out excess liquid and mucus from the lungs.

Ingredients:

2 cups, or 1 long lotus root, sliced thin diagonally
¼ tsp sea salt, or to taste
A generous pinch of cumin or mango powder (amchur)
1½ tbsp oil for pan-frying

Method:

1. Lightly steam the lotus root for 1–2 minutes and set aside
    to dry off.
2. In a ceramic or Le Creuset flat skillet, heat 1 tbsp oil and
    pan-fry the lotus slices on both sides on a low flame until
    light brown.
3. Wipe the pan clean with a paper towel between batches as
    the oil gets hot. Add a dash more of the oil and continue
    to pan-fry.
4. Add salt and mango powder to taste. Serve hot.

Sweet Potato Tikkis

This recipe serves 4–5 people.

Ingredients:

1 large sweet potato, boiled, peeled and mashed
1 organic regular potato, boiled, peeled and mashed
1 tsp mango powder (amchur)
½ tsp sea salt, or to taste
Organic cold-pressed sesame oil, or organic ghee

Method:

1. Mix all the ingredients and make patties. Pan-fry on both sides on a medium–low flame until light brown.
2. Serve hot with coriander–mint or coriander–mango chutney.

Lotus and Vegetable Stir-fry

This is a simple yet dynamic dish. We first sauté thin matchstick cut vegetables and then allow these to simmer for 12–15 minutes. The act of first actively sautéing these and then simmering them gives us the same energy, that is, active (like actively stirring and sautéing) and then, rested strong energy (like simmering) at the same time. This is a great dish for people who have a lot of work to do as it gives them 'pick-up' and active energy!

Ingredients:

1½ cup carrots, cut like matchsticks
½ cup green beans, cut into 2-inch pieces
2 cups or 2 medium–small onions, cut into half-moons
1–1½ tbsp ginger juice from freshly grated ginger
1 green chilli, de-seeded and cut into small pieces (optional)
½ tsp sea salt, or to taste
1 tbsp organic or tamari (high-quality wheat-free) soy sauce
2 tsp toasted sesame oil

Method:

1. Heat oil in a stainless steel skillet and add the onions and green chilli with ¼ tsp salt. Sauté for 1–2 minutes and lower the flame. Cover the base of the pan. Layer the carrots and the beans on top of the carrots. Add enough water to cover just the onions. Turn up the flame for a minute until the water bubbles. Then lower the flame and cook covered for 10–12 minutes or until the vegetables are well-cooked (not overcooked) and there is no more water.
2. Add salt or tamari to taste. Stir in the ginger juice and turn off the flame. Serve hot.

Tips and Variations:

1. Do not add the ginger juice until just before serving. If you add the ginger juice and re-heat later, there will be little flavour left.
2. You may add lotus root to the above dish.

Bitter Gourd Subzi

Bitter gourd is a blood cleanser that also detoxifies the lungs and the heart. It also helps maintain healthy blood sugar levels.

Ingredients:

4 cups or 5 medium bitter gourds, cut into thin circles with 2 flat tsp sea salt rubbed in for an hour before cooking
2–2½ cups or 2 medium–small onions, cut into thin quarter-moons
1½ tbsp tamarind, soaked in ½ cup water for 30 minutes

2½ tbsp powdered jaggery
2–3 tbsp organic cold-pressed sesame oil
½ tsp sea salt

Method:

1. Heat 1 tbsp oil in a ceramic or Le Crueset flat or shallow pan. Add the bitter gourd and cook on medium–low heat for 3–4 minutes. Turn the side and cook for another 3–4 minutes on the other side. Add oil if needed. Cook to desired crunchiness.
2. In a separate stainless steel skillet, heat the oil and add the onions with ½ tsp salt. Sauté for 1–2 minutes.
3. Mush and mix the tamarind in the soaking water and strain, saving the liquid.
4. Add the tamarind liquid and jaggery to the onions and sauté on low heat for 1–2 minutes. Stir in the bitter gourd and adjust the seasoning (sweet and sour flavours) and salt to taste. Serve hot.

Coconut Vegetable Stew

This is a sweet and rich vegetable dish. It has a relaxing effect on the lungs and kidneys.

This recipe serves 3–4 people.

Ingredients:

½ cup carrots, cut into thin quarter-moon slices or small cubes
½ cup white radish, cut into thin quarter-moon slices or small cubes
½ cup green beans, cut small into 1-inch pieces
½ cup or 1 medium-small onion, cut into quarter-moon slices or small cubes

½ cup snap peas, cut diagonally
½ red small bell pepper, de-seeded and cut into thin slices
1 cup or ¼ small sweet potato, cut into small cubes
1½ cup fresh mushrooms of your choice, wiped with a clean kitchen towel
1 tbsp ginger, minced
1 tbsp or 3–4 garlic cloves, crushed or minced
2–3 green chillies, de-seeded and cut small
½ tsp ground turmeric
A pinch of black pepper
½ cup fresh basil leaves, hard stems removed, roughly chopped
1 drop high-grade organic lemongrass oil
1–1½ tsp powdered jaggery, or to taste (start with less and add more if needed)
½–1 tbsp fresh lemon juice, or to taste
2 cups organic unsweetened coconut milk, freshly pressed at home or bought organic

Method:

1. Heat oil in a large stainless steel skillet or wok. Add the onions with a pinch of salt and sauté for 1–2 minutes. Stir in the ginger and garlic and cook for another minute. Slowly stir in all other vegetables, except the peppers and snap peas. Mix well and add a dash of water if needed. Lower the flame and simmer for 1–2 minutes, leaving the vegetables slightly crunchy.

2. Stir in ½–¾ cup water and the coconut cream. Bring to a gentle boil. Add the peppers, snap peas, powdered jaggery, lemongrass oil and salt to taste. Simmer for another 1–2 minutes.

3. Add the lime or lemon juice and chopped fresh basil just before serving.

Tips and Variations:

1. The quality of coconut cream differs according to brands and countries. Hence the quantity of salt, sweet and lemon may have to be adjusted as per the variety you use.

Stir-Fried Vegetables

This recipe serves 2–3 people.

Ingredients:

1 cup or 1 medium onion, cut into half-moons
1 cup or 1 large carrot, halved lengthwise and sliced into thin diagonals
1½ cups lotus root or 1 lotus root, halved and cut into thin diagonals
1 cup snap peas, cut diagonally
1 cup broccoli florets, steamed
2–2½ tsp toasted sesame oil
1¼ tbsp ginger juice squeezed from freshly grated ginger
2–3 cloves of garlic, pressed or minced
1–2 tsp high-grade or organic tamari to taste (optional)
½ tsp sea salt, or to taste

Method:

1. In a heavy based stainless steel pan, heat 1½ tsp oil and add the onions with a pinch of salt. Sauté for about a minute. Add the garlic and all the vegetables (harder vegetables first) and sauté for a few minutes until cooked. Remember to leave them a little crunchy. Add water if needed.

2. Add the tamari, ginger juice, ½ tsp toasted sesame oil and salt. Cook for another 30 seconds. Mix well and serve hot over rice or noodles.

Tips and Variations:

1. You may steam the vegetables and let them dry before you sauté them for just a minute. This will avoid any chances of burning or breaking the vegetables from over stirring. It also uses less oil.

2. You may sauté the vegetables or a single vegetable in olive oil with a pinch of salt and garlic if you wish. For example, sautéed broccoli and bok choy.

Quick Sautéed Leeks

This recipe serves 2–3 people.

Ingredients:

2 large leeks, halved lengthwise and washed and cut diagonally
2 tsp organic cold-pressed sesame oil or organic cold-pressed olive oil
A generous pinch of sea salt, or to taste
A dash of lemon (optional)

Method:

1. Heat oil in a stainless steel or ceramic pan. Add the leeks and a generous pinch of sea salt. Sauté for 2–3 minutes. Serve hot.

Simple Indian-Style cauliflower

Ginger, turmeric, black pepper and cauliflower have a cleansing effect on the alveoli. They help to remove stagnated blood and toxic buildup in the lungs.

This recipe serves two people.

Ingredients:

2½–3 cups cauliflower florets
¼–½ sweet peas
½ tsp ground turmeric
½ tsp ground cumin (optional)
A pinch of freshly ground black pepper
1½ tbsp ginger, minced or cut very thin
2 tsp salt, or to taste
½ cup fresh cilantro, for garnishing
2 tsp cold-pressed organic sesame oil and 1 tsp organic ghee, or 3 tsp organic cold-pressed sesame oil

Method:

1. Heat oil in a stainless steel pan. Add the ginger and sauté for a minute. Add the sweet peas and then the cauliflower with turmeric, cumin, salt and a little water. Lower the flame and cook for 10–12 minutes until the vegetables are well-cooked.
2. Turn off the flame, sprinkle with black pepper and stir well. Garnish and serve hot.

Tips and Variations:

1. You may use whole cumin seeds instead of ground cumin.
2. You may add 1–2 de-seeded green chilies.
3. You can sprinkle a pinch of garam masala along with the black pepper before serving.

19

Essential Salads

Salads are an essential part of every meal, but are often ignored. They offer nourishing and relaxing energy. If a person does not consume salads often, their system may feel heavy and sluggish. In fact, this is true for both healthy alkalinity-promoting soups and salads. They aid digestion and assimilation of other healthy foods.

Here are some recipes that are extremely beneficial:

1. Grated White Radish Salad (page 186)
2. Steamed or Blanched Salad (page 187)
3. Wholesome Salad (page 188)
4. Mixed Sprouts Salad (page 189)

Grated White Radish Salad

White radish is a root vegetable associated with the element of metal. Incidentally, white is the colour of metal. Lungs too are related to the element of metal which makes this salad an excellent option to melt mucus buildup in the digestive organs as well as the lungs.

I recommend that you have around 2 tbsp of this salad at least three to four times a week when in season.

This recipe serves 2 people.

Ingredients:

1 large white radish or 1 cup packed grated white radish (mooli)
½ tsp high-grade maple syrup or organic raw honey
1½ tbsp freshly squeezed lemon juice
¼ tsp of sea salt
1 tbsp fresh coriander/cilantro or parsley leaves, roughly cut, for garnishing

Method:

1. Place the grated white radish in a glass bowl.
2. Mix the maple/honey, lemon juice and salt in a separate bowl. Pour this over the white radish and mix well. Add fresh coriander/cilantro/parsley and mix well. Serve cool.

Tips and Variations:

1. You can add 1 tsp of home-made spiced mustard dip for a more pungent flavour.
2. You may add some carrots to add colour to this salad.

Steamed or Blanched Salad

Ideally, a person should consume at least one helping of steamed or blanched vegetables every day. Choose root, round and leafy green vegetables and steam them to desired crunchiness. For blanching, boil water and add a pinch of salt and dip the vegetables for 30–90 seconds depending on the vegetable. Pull out using a blanching stick. Generally, green vegetables should remain bright green whether steamed or blanched. Overcooking vegetables leads them to lose the bright colour.

For stronger lungs, choose these vegetables: lotus root, broccoli, cauliflower, white radish, carrots, red radish, leeks, zucchini, bottle or round gourd and dark leafy greens such as bathua, spinach, mustard greens, radish greens and kale. You can also opt for calcium-rich greens such as bok choy, cabbage, Brussels sprouts, etc. Occasionally, you can use these vegetables: sweet potatoes, beetroot, okra, pumpkin, etc.

Wholesome Salad

You can have 2–3 cups of this salad with every meal.

Ingredients:

You can use easy-to-digest raw vegetables such as cucumbers, lettuce, zucchini and salad greens of your choice. Restrain from consuming vegetables like broccoli, carrots and cauliflowers raw as these are difficult to digest.

Method:

1. Steam or blanch the vegetables of your choice.
2. Add toasted, unsweetened seeds or nuts of your choice, whole or broken into 2–3 pieces each. For example, toasted sesame seeds, sunflower seeds, flax seeds, walnuts, almonds, cashews, peanuts, etc.

3. Add sprouts and microgreens (alfafa sprouts, fenugreek sprouts, broccoli sprouts, radish sprouts, etc.) for extra nutrition.
4. Add avocados, or steamed sweet potatoes, beetroot, gooseberries (amla), cranberries, olives, capers for varied flavour.
5. Add noodles, amaranth, quinoa, barley, etc., for variety.
6. Add a high-quality organic apple–cider vinegar or lemon juice, or choose a dressing of your choice.

Tips and Variations:

1. You can combine raw zucchini, raw cucumbers, iceberg lettuce, beetroot microgreens, steamed or raw carrots (if using raw carrots, cut them paper-thin).
2. You can use steamed lotus root, broccoli, bottle gourd, bok choy, snap peas, sprouts and toasted sesame seeds.
3. You may also use lettuce, salad greens, cucumbers, steamed or baked sweet potato (cubed or sliced), toasted walnuts, toasted sesame seeds.
4. Raw baby spinach, lettuce, cucumbers, fenugreek sprouts, steamed broccoli, alfafa sprouts are also good options.

Mixed Sprout Salad

This recipe serves 2 people.

Ingredients:

1 cup moong bean sprouts, raw or lightly steamed as per your choice
¾ cup alfalfa sprouts

½ cup broccoli sprouts (optional)
½ cup radish sprouts
¼ cup fenugreek sprouts
½ cup spring onions/scallions or shallots, cut small (optional)
1½–2 cups cucumber, cut very small (to match the size of the sprouts) and steamed
Fresh lemon juice to taste
A generous pinch of sea salt to taste

Method:

1. Mix all the ingredients in a bowl. Add lemon and salt, and serve fresh.

Tips and Variations:

1. Add fresh coriander or fresh parsley leaves as garnish.
2. Add one de-seeded green chilli to the salad.
3. You may also add bean sprouts, for example, sprouts made from moth bean (matki), brown chickpeas and horse gram lentil.

20

Alkalizing Oil-free Pickles and Condiments

Pickles traditionally served the purpose of digesting a meal better. Some pickles also added good flavour to a meal. The fermentation provide good bacteria to the stomach and gut thereby aiding digestion. Not just this, but fermented foods also help improve our immunity.

Home-made pickles are usually better than those available commercially. The only exception to this rule is when the person making it at home uses toxic ingredients unknowingly or for convenience. Remember, a few pieces of oil-free fermented pickle a day will keep the doctor away.

What kinds of pickles are detrimental to our digestion and immunity?

1. Pickles that are made using poor-quality oil or refined oils.
2. Pickles that are made with excessive oil.
3. Most market-bought pickles that have preservatives and chemicals.
4. Most market-bought pickles that have artificial food colours.

5. Pickles that are made with excessive spices and garlic as these can overstimulate the digestive and nervous systems.

How to Make a Pickle?

The amount of vegetables and pickling liquid you use will depend on the size of the jar you use. I begin by filling up an empty and dry glass jar with the vegetable and then adding the pickling liquid. You may need to use another jar or use more vegetables or pickling liquid as per your requirement. Don't use plastic jars for pickles. You can use the method below for most pickles here, except the lemon pickle and sauerkraut.

After this, take 1–2 cabbage leaves, cover the vegetables and press them down so that the vegetables and the cabbage leaves are below the picking liquid. Cover the jar with cheesecloth or thin white muslin cloth (use a string or a rubber band to secure the cloth). Leave it in a cool, dark place for 25–35 hours (about 1½ days). Remove the cabbage leaves and any froth that may have formed, and then cover and refrigerate. The pickle will be ready in 2–3 days.

Sauerkraut takes up to 10–14 days to be ready. You should check it every 1–2 days and change the cabbage leaf (with clean hands) every 2–3 days. Remove any excess froth that may form. It is important to note that pickles should be made in a glass jar or non-reactive ceramic jars. Never use plastic, metal or other reactive containers.

Carrot–Radish Pickle

Ingredients:

1 cup carrots, cut like matchsticks
3 cups white radish, cut like matchsticks
2 bay leaves

Pickling liquid:

3½–4 cups water
1½–2 tbsp sea salt to taste
4 black peppercorns
2–3 cloves of garlic, crushed
½ cup brown rice vinegar or natural apple cider vinegar
1½–2 tbsp powdered jaggery diluted in a little water, or 1 tbsp
high-grade pure maple syrup

Traditional Brine Pickle

Ingredients:

2 cups organic white cabbage, shredded
1–2 cup carrots, cut like matchsticks

Pickling liquid:

4 cups water
2¼ tbsp sea salt

Sauerkraut

Ingredients:

1 large head cabbage
2 tsp caraway seeds (optional)
1–1¼ tbsp sea salt, or to taste

Method:

Shred the cabbage and place it in a large glass or stainless
steel bowl. Massage the salt into the vegetables for about
8–12 minutes or until it releases some liquid. Transfer it to

a medium–large wide-mouth glass jar. Take 1–2 cabbage leaves and cover the vegetables. Press them down so that the vegetables and the cabbage leaves are below the picking liquid. Unlike other pickles, no pickling liquid is added here. The only liquid here is released from the cabbage. Cover the jar with cheesecloth or a thin white muslin cloth (use a string or a rubber band to secure the cloth) and then leave in a cool dark place for 10–12 days (Given the tropical weather in New Delhi, I usually make mine in 10 days). You should check it every 1–2 days and change the cabbage leaf (with clean hands) every two days. Remove any excess froth that may form.

Once it is ready, remove the froth and the cabbage leaf. Cover and refrigerate. Have 1–2 tsp with meals every day. If you are making a large quantity, you may use a ceramic pickling pot and place a glass plate on it. You can then place a heavy stone (about 1½–2 kg, or 5 pounds) and press it down so that the liquid is above the level of the plate.

If making sauerkraut in a place that has humid and hot weather, there may be a lot of froth that will have to be removed every 8–10 hours. Also, the cabbage leaf will have to be changed every day (if you are using in a jar). Sometimes, in such weather conditions, sauerkraut may even be ready in 3–5 days. This will be more like a quick pickle than the traditional sauerkraut. I usually avoid making sauerkraut in the rainy season and prefer simple brine or umeboshi pickles instead.

Haldi Pickle

Ingredients:

About 2 cups raw, whole turmeric root, peeled and cut like matchsticks

Pickling liquid:

½-3/4 cup lemon juice
1 cup water
1 tbsp sea salt

Lemon Pickle

Ingredients:

5 kg organic lemons, rinsed, dried, cut into quarters with the whole peel and partially or fully de-seeded.
220–250 gm sea salt

Method:

Cut the lemons into half or bite-size pieces. Rub the salt and seasoning in and place in a dry glass jar. Cover and tie up with layers of cloth to prevent any moisture from entering. Place this jar in the sun for 2 hours every day for 10–12 days and then place it in the shade for the rest of the day. After 10–12 days, leave it indoors for another 2–3 months. With time, the lemon peel becomes soft and loses its bitterness. My grandmother usually made this pickle in November and it was ready for use in spring and summer.

Tips and Variations:

1. Some people add only salt, while others add salt, turmeric, carom seeds, fenugreek seeds, cumin and very little garam masala. All these spices are used in powdered form.

Condiments

Just like pickles, condiments too can be beneficial or harmful. Home-made condiments with mineral-rich seeds, nuts and sea salt are less likely to do any harm while commercial condiments contain chemicals and excitotoxins.

MSG is an excitotoxin that leads to nerve damage and neuro-degenerative disorders. It is often added to Chinese food and is used at many commercial restaurants. Even if it is not directly added to a dish, it is often part of bottled sauces that are used for cooking. Phrases like 'natural flavourings', 'high in energy', 'real ingredients' can be misleading and deceiving.

Home-made Sesame Seed Salt

This is an alkalizing condiment that is good for asthmatics and aids digestion. You can use 1 tsp a day over grains such as rice, barley, millets, etc. You will need a suribachi, or a mortar and pestle, for this recipe.

Ingredients:

22 tbsp tan or black sesame seeds
1 tbsp high-quality sea salt
Suribachi or mortar and pestle

Method:

1. Rinse the sesame seeds and roast them on a wide stainless steel skillet over a medium flame. Stir continuously with a wooden or bamboo spoon. As the seeds begin to dry,

within 30–90 seconds, lower the flame and continue stirring, ensuring that all seeds get equal heat. Don't stop stirring as it may burn some seeds. When the seeds are done, in about 5–7 minutes, transfer them to the mortar and pestle. To check if the seeds are done, pick up a few of them with a dry spoon. If they stick to the spoon, they are not done. Also, they should begin to give out a fragrance if they are done. You can also crush a seed between your fingers to check if it is crunchy. Make sure the seeds are not overdone. To ensure this is the case, roast the seeds on a low flame except for the first 1–1½ minutes.

2. Roast the sea salt for about a minute and add to the mortar and pestle.

3. Grind while both are hot until the seeds are 70 per cent crushed. Store in a dry glass jar and keep in a cool dark place. This home-made sesame seed salt can be stored for up to 2–3 weeks.

Tips and Variations:

1. You may add 2 tbsp roasted jeera to this recipe.
2. If making a large quantity, you may use a mixer grinder.
3. You may add small quantities of any combination of these nuts or seeds during the grinding process in the end: toasted sunflower seeds or peanuts, dried coconut powder or toasted flax seeds.

21

Nutritious Dips and Dressings

This chapter lists out some flavourful dips that can add the extra zing to your salads or any other meal.

1. Basil–Pine Nut Dressing (page 199)
2. Curry Leaf–Sesame Chutney (page 199)
3. Peanut Chutney (page 200)
4. Indian Cranberry Chutney (Karonde) (page 201)
5. Home-made Mustard Spread (page 202)
6. Home-made Mustard Marinade (page 203)
7. Carrot–Almond Dressing (page 203)
8. Orange–Lemon Dressing (page 204)
9. Tahini–Lemon Dressing (page 205)
10. Sweet and Sour Peanut Butter Dressing (page 206)
11. Raw Mango–Cilantro Chutney (page 206)
12. Coriander–Mint Chutney (page 207)
13. Sweet-Gingery Sesame Dressing (page 208)
14. Tamarind Sauce (page 209)
15. Guacamole (Avocado dip) (page 210)

Basil–Pine Nut Dressing

Leafy greens nourish the lungs, heart and the liver. Basil is known to be anti-microbial, anti-inflammatory and rich in antioxidants. Basil leaves help reduce the risk of infections and improve the immune function. Organic or home-grown leaves, without pesticides, are even more beneficial.

Ingredients:

2–2½ packed cups basil, washed and hard stems removed
1 tbsp powdered jaggery, or ¾ tbsp high-grade maple syrup, or 1 tbsp brown rice nectar
2½–3 tbsp fresh lemon juice, or to taste
2–3 cloves/2–3 tsp garlic, crushed or pressed
¼ cup pine nuts, lightly toasted on a medium–low flame for 2–4 minutes
18–20 cashews
¾ tsp sea salt, or to taste
⅙–¼ cup water

Method:

1. Grind all ingredients to a smooth consistency.

Tips and Variations:

1. Store pine nuts in the refrigerator as these can attract ants if left out. This depends on the climate where you live.

Curry Leaf–Sesame Chutney

Curry leaves and sesame seeds are rich in calcium, magnesium, iron and other minerals and support the healing process. I recommend having a teaspoon four to six times a week.

Ingredients:

1 cup packed fresh curry leaves, de-stemmed
2 tbsp tamarind, soaked in ½ cup water for 30 minutes
3 tbsp unseasoned toasted sesame seeds
1–1½ tsp powdered jaggery
1 large clove of garlic, pressed or minced
2 tsp ginger, minced
¼ tsp sea salt, or to taste
½ small green chilli, de-seeded and cut small
Pinch of black pepper

Method:

1. Mix the tamarind pulp with the soaking water and strain, saving the liquid. Use this liquid while blending.
2. Take the tamarind-flavoured liquid, curry leaves, powdered jaggery and salt and blend until smooth. Add all the other ingredients and blend again. Adjust the salt and sweet flavours to taste.

Peanut Chutney

This is a delicious addition to any meal. Use sparingly as it has tomatoes.

Ingredients:

¼ cup unsalted shelled peanuts
3 medium tomatoes, cut small

1 medium onion, cut very small
6–8 cloves garlic, minced
1 tsp ginger, minced
½–1 tsp sea salt, or to taste
1 tsp organic ghee or organic cold-pressed sesame oil
½–1 cup water

Method:

1. Rinse and toast the peanuts on a medium–low flame for 7–10 minutes until fragrant and toasted, but not burnt. Set aside to cool.
2. In a stainless steel saucepan, heat the ghee or oil. Add the onion with a pinch of salt. Sauté for a minute. Add the garlic, ginger, tomatoes and salt. Sauté stirring occasionally on a low flame. Add ¼–½ cup of water and cook covered for 3–5 minutes. Turn off the flame and let it cool.
3. Once everything has cooled down, grind in a mixer, adding water and salt to the desired level of consistency and taste. Serve at room temperature and refrigerate for future use.

Tips and Variations:

1. You may also add 2 tbsp lightly roasted hemp seeds (bhang) to this recipe. Adjust/increase other ingredients marginally. Bhang seeds are traditionally used in peanut chutney in the mountain regions of India. Hemp cannabis seeds are not intoxicating or illegal like other parts of the plant.

Indian Cranberry Chutney

Therapeutic and anti-inflammatory, this chutney also helps improve blood circulation.

Ingredients:

½ cup Indian cranberries (karonde), cut into half lengthwise
1 packed cup fresh coriander/cilantro leaves
2 large green chillies, de-seeded (the larger ones are less spicy.
Start with one and add more if needed)
1 tbsp toasted sesame seeds
1 tsp ginger, minced
1 tsp lemon juice (optional and to taste)
1 tsp powdered jaggery (optional)
¼ tsp sea salt, or to taste
2 tbsp water

Method:

1. Blend all the ingredients to the desired consistency.
   Adjust salt to taste.

Home-made Mustard Spread

Good-quality mustard used in moderation has a therapeutic
effect on the lungs. This home-made mustard spread tastes
better after being refrigerated for a week or two, as it becomes
more gentle and less sharp in flavour. You may add a little of
this to salad dressings and other dips for a pungent flavour.

Ingredients:

3 tbsp large yellow mustard seeds, soaked for 6–8 hours
2 tbsp large black mustard seeds, soaked for 6–8 hours
2 tsp ginger, minced
1–2 tsp garlic, minced to taste

2 tbsp powdered jaggery or any organic natural sweetener of choice to taste (you can opt for organic raw honey or brown rice nectar)
2 tbsp fresh lemon juice
¼ tsp sea salt
1 tbsp mustard oil
¼–½ cup water (if you add more water, the seasoning may have to be adjusted accordingly)
A pinch of black pepper

Method:

1. Grind to a creamy, smooth paste in a small grinder. If the blender is too large, the paste may remain course. Store in the refrigerator for up to 7–10 days.

Tips and Variations:

1. The ginger should be well minced so that the fibrous part does not stay unmixed.

Home-made Mustard Marinade (for fish)

When marinating a fish with this, don't use the whole marinade. Use some and keep a little for adding just before serving the fish.

I add a teaspoon of cumin seeds and two teaspoons of carom seeds to the home-made mustard spread and blend it all to make a smooth paste.

Carrot–Almond Dressing

A delicious and creamy yet light dressing that goes well with blanched and boiled vegetables.

Ingredients:

¾ cup or 1 medium carrot, cubed
1–1½ tbsp pure unsweetened organic almond butter
1 tsp ginger, minced
1 tsp garlic minced
½ tsp rice vinegar
1¼ tsp toasted sesame oil
1–1½ tbsp fresh lemon juice, or to taste
¼ tsp sea salt
½ cup water

Method:

1. Blend all ingredients to make a thick, yet creamy, smooth paste.

Orange–Lemon Dressing

A light and refreshing traditional olive oil-based salad dressing.

Ingredients:

¾ cup fresh orange or kinnow juice
1 clove of garlic, crushed
2 tbsp olive oil
¾ tsp sea salt, or to taste
¼ tsp black pepper
1 tsp lemon juice
½ tsp maple syrup (optional)

Method:

1. Whisk all the ingredients in a glass jar and shake well.

Tahini-Lemon Dressing

An all-time favourite with most people. Sometimes, when the dressing is delicious, people have more salads and greens.

Ingredients:

½ cup tahini
3 tbsp lemon juice
¼ tsp sea salt
1–1½ tsp powdered jaggery, or high-grade maple syrup, or brown rice nectar (start with 1 tbsp and add more if required)
1 cup water

Method:

1. Blend all ingredients with a cup of water. Adjust sweet and lemon to taste.

Tips and Variations:

1. Keep the dressing on the thinner side as it thickens with time.
2. You can add fresh dill, parsley, spring onions/scallions or mint for a different flavour. If adding spring onions/scallions, then it must be consumed within 24–30 hours.
3. You may also add a dash of the home-made mustard spread for a creamy mustard dressing.

Sweet and Sour Peanut Butter Dressing

This goes well with salads, noodles and steamed vegetables.

Ingredients:

2 tbsp organic unsweetened peanut butter
¼ cup water or to desired consistency
1 tsp or 1–2 cloves of garlic, minced
2 tsp ginger, minced
2 tsp jaggery or 1½–2 tsp of any natural sweetener of your choice (organic honey or maple syrup)
¼ tsp salt
1 tbsp lemon juice

Method:

1. Blend all ingredients until creamy and smooth. Adjust sweetener, lemon and water to desired consistency and taste. Serve over a salad or greens.

Tips and Variations:

1. You may add fresh cilantro and a little mint for a more fragrant taste.
2. Buy peanut butter without oil, refined sugars and preservatives.

Raw Mango-Cilantro Chutney

A delicious tangy dressing for occasional use. Do not use if your condition is very sensitive.

Ingredients:

1½ packed cups of fresh coriander/cilantro leaves, rinsed and roughly cut
1 tbsp and 1 tsp powdered jaggery, or to taste
¼ cup or one medium–small raw mango
¼ tsp ground coriander
¼ tsp sea salt, or to taste
1 tbsp mint leaves

Method:

1. Blend all ingredients and adjust the seasoning to taste. Serve chilled with khichdi, lemon quinoa, sweet potato patties, croquettes, rice congee or kala chana kebabs, etc.

Tips and Variations:

1. If you have a high inflammatory and sensitive condition, then you may omit the mango and make coriander–mint chutney (see below).

Coriander–Mint chutney

Coriander/cilantro leaves and mint have a cleansing effect on the lungs. Ginger and lemon juice cut through excess mucus buildup in the lungs.

I recommend having this three to four times a week.

Ingredients:

2 packed cups fresh coriander/cilantro leaves
¾ cup fresh mint leaves, hard stems removed

2 tbsp lemon juice

1–½ tsp powdered jaggery, or to taste (start with 1 tsp and add more if needed)

2–3 tbsp water (start with less and add a maximum of ¼ cup water)

2 tbsp spring onions/scallion or leeks, cut fine (use the white part)

¼ tsp sea salt, or to taste

Method:

1. Blend all ingredients to desired consistency. Add salt and lemon to taste. Serve with lemon quinoa, rice dishes, croquettes, patties/tikkis, etc. You can store this in a glass jar and keep it in the refrigerator for up to 3–5 days.

Tips and Variations:

1. If your health permits, then you may add 1 de-seeded green chilli.
2. You can also try the amla–coriander–mint chutney. All you need to do is add one grated amla to the recipe above.

Sweet–Gingery Sesame Dressing

An Asian-style dressing which is great over steamed or crunchy raw salads, stir-fried vegetable dishes, noodles and other grain-based salads.

Ingredients:

2½–3 tbsp toasted sesame oil

2 tbsp high-grade maple syrup

1 tbsp ginger juice
2 tbsp lemon juice
1 tbsp tamari
1 tbsp fresh spring onions or fresh cilantro, or to taste

Method:

1.   Mix all ingredients with a whisk and serve cool.

Tamarind Sauce

This sauce goes well with steamed white radish. It also goes well with grains and boiled sweet potatoes or other root vegetables.

Ingredients:

2 tbsp peeled tamarind, soaked in ½ cup water for 30–60 minutes
2½–2 tsp powdered jaggery, or to taste
1/2 tsp arrowroot or kudzu diluted in 2 tbsp water
½ tsp sea salt

Method:

1.   Mix the soaked tamarind and strain the seeds and fibre out, leaving behind a thick paste.
2.   Add this, the powdered jaggery, salt and the diluted arrowroot to a stainless steel skillet and cook on a medium–low flame. As it begins to boil, lower the flame and let it thicken. As the arrowroot thickens and loosens its whiteness, the sauce is ready. Adjust the salt and sour and sweet flavours to taste. Serve over steamed white radish or your choice of steamed vegetables.

Guacamole

A delicious creamy dip that goes well with a bean wrap or veggie sticks. Use sparingly, and in moderation, if your condition is very sensitive.

Ingredients:

3 large avocados, mashed (add ¾ tsp lemon juice to keep it from turning dark)
Lemon juice to taste
½ cup onion or spring onions/scallions, minced
2 tbsp fresh coriander/cilantro leaves
½ tsp sea salt or umeboshi paste, or to taste

Method:

1. Mix all the ingredients in a bowl. Add salt and lemon to taste. Serve with beans and corn tortillas.

22

Healthy Snacks and Desserts

Snacks should be consumed in very small quantities at one time while desserts should not be had more than twice a week.

Besides the list on the next page, all small quantities of left-over dishes like fried polenta, millet croquettes, brown rice tikkis, red rice poha, lemon quinoa also make for good snacks. If your digestion is weak, or if you are prone to fatigue, you should have small servings of snacks at one time.

This section also includes recipes for desserts, which should be used sparingly and in moderation during the healing phase. After one's blood quality and condition has improved, then one can have desserts occasionally to maintain and sustain good health. It is always beneficial to have a hot, healing or home-made herbal tea along with or within ½–1 hour of consuming any sweet snack or desserts. The hot, sugar-free, and often alkalizing or soothing, tea after desserts also helps keep the organs functioning with efficiency. Consuming anything in excess and without the right combination may lead to blood stagnation or affect one's digestion. Moderation is key when making and consuming desserts. Here are some of the recipes:

Sunflower Seed Trail Mix

This is a traditional trail mix that uses nuts, seeds and dried fruits. You can have this in small quantities (1–2 tbsp) as a snack if you feel hungry between meals.

Ingredients:

¾ cup toasted sunflower seeds (175°C for 12–15 minutes)
2 tbsp black raisins
¼ cup toasted almonds (175°C for 8–12 minutes)
1 tbsp chopped, unsweetened dried apricots
6–8 toasted walnuts, each walnut broken into 2–3 pieces
4–5 raw cashews, each cashew cut into 2–3 pieces

Method:

1. Mix and store in an airtight glass container in the refrigerator.

Lemony Mashed Sweet Potatoes

This recipe serves two people.

Ingredients:

1 medium sweet potato, boiled, peeled and mashed
Lemon juice to taste
A generous pinch of sea salt or Himalayan pink salt
2–3 tbsp unsalted roasted peanuts
2 tbsp fresh coriander/cilantro leaves, for garnishing

Method:

1. Add lemon juice and salt to taste. Try to use less salt as this dish is relaxing for the organs when sweet and lemony with just a tad bit of salt.
2. Sprinkle with toasted peanuts and garnish and serve warm or at room temperature.

Apricot Kanten

Kanten is a relaxing dessert. It helps to relax contractions in the lungs during an attack and, unlike commercial Jell-O, it is made of a sea vegetable called agar-agar which is a good source of calcium and iron.

Ingredients:

4 cups organic unsweetened apple juice
1–2 small apricots, sliced thin, or 1 cup cantaloupe, cubed
4–5 blueberries or cherries de-seeded and halved, or any berry of choice
4 tbsp kanten flakes
A few petals of an edible flower (optional)
1 tbsp organic, aluminium-free arrowroot powder or kudzu root powder, diluted in 2 tbsp cold water
¼ tsp sea salt
2–3 tbsp powdered jaggery, or maple syrup, or brown rice syrup
2 tbsp fresh lemon juice (optional, and good in the summer time)

Method:

1. Add the kanten flakes to the apple juice and let it sit covered for 30–45 minutes. This ensures that there are no lumps later. If you are using powdered jaggery, then you should add it now.
2. Add the well-diluted arrowroot or kudzu root. Stir well before heating.
3. Heat on a medium–low flame, stirring constantly with a bamboo or wooden flat spoon for about 5–8 minutes. Once it comes to a gentle boil, turn off the flame.
4. If you are not adding jaggery, then add the maple or rice syrup now and mix well. Stir in the lemon juice.
5. Put the cut fruit into a large glass bowl or individual dessert cups and add the hot juice mix over it. You could also pour the kanten mix into a bowl and decorate with sliced apricots. After 10–15 minutes, add the cherries and

flower petals. Refrigerate for up to two hours or until it sets like Jell-O.

Tips and Variations:

1. You may add any fruit of your choice such as berries, pears, apples, etc.

Puffed Rice and Amaranth Snack

A light puffed oil-free snack for occasional use.

Ingredients:

1½ cups puffed rice
1½ cups puffed amaranth
2–3 tbsp roasted peanuts
1½ tbsp roasted flax seeds
2–3 tbsp roasted sunflower seeds
½ tsp sea salt or to taste
¼ tsp powdered jaggery (optional)
20–25 curry leaves
¾ tsp roasted ground cumin
A generous pinch of garlic powder
A pinch of ground black pepper

Method:

1. Wash and lightly roast (without oil) the curry leaves for 2–3 minutes, or until they begin to dry, on a medium–low flame. Add the puffed rice and roast for another 1–2 minutes.

2. Transfer into a glass bowl and mix in the seasoning. Store
    in an airtight jar.

Tips and Variations:

1. Rinse and roast the sunflower seeds and peanuts at 300°F
    or 150°C for 12–15 minutes.

Roasted Lotus Seeds (Makhane)

All parts of the lotus plant are therapeutic for the lungs.
Lightly puffed and toasted lotus seeds make for a healthy
and light snack. Eat this in moderation as it is as delicious
as buttered popcorn, making it easy for anyone to
overeat.

Ingredients:

3 cups puffed lotus seeds
½–1 tsp sea salt, or to taste
1–2 tsp organic ghee (optional)

Method:

1. Roast the puffed lotus seeds on a medium–low flame for
    about 5–7 minutes, or until crunchy.
2. Add the salt and stir in the ghee. Turn off the heat.
3. Mix well and store in an airtight glass jar.

Sweet Potato Chips

This is a delicious dish to add variety to your cooking.

Ingredients:

2 sweet potatoes or yams, peeled and cut into half or quarter-moon slices
2 tbsp coconut oil or high-grade cold-pressed olive oil (do not use pure or pomace olive oil)
2 tsp ground cumin
1½ tsp sea salt, or to taste

Method:

1. Pre-heat the oven to 180°C.
2. Mix all ingredients in a bowl. Place them on a parchment paper and bake for about twenty minutes, or until crisp and lightly brown.

Tips and Variations:

1. Each oven and the variety of sweet potatoes or yams used is different. Watch closely to adjust cooking time. Turn off the oven if the dish seems brown on one side and not the other.

Home-made Granola Bar

This granola bar has no white sugar, no oil, no chemicals or preservatives. It is made with fresh ingredients and is packed with wholesome nutrition.

Ingredients:

1 cup pitted dates, roughly chopped
1 cup oat flakes, toasted in the oven for 15 minutes at 180°C

1 cup almonds, toasted in the oven for 8–10 minutes at 150°C, roughly chopped
¼ cup sunflower seeds, toasted in the oven for 12–14 minutes at 150°C, roughly chopped
2 tbsp lightly toasted flax seeds, toast on a dry skillet on medium–low heat for 3–5 minutes, stirring continuously (you could also buy toasted flax seeds)
1/3 cup smooth almond butter
1–2 tbsp high-grade maple syrup, or to taste
1½ tsp organic vanilla extract
Pinch of sea salt
Pinch of ground cinnamon

Method:

1. Mix all the ingredients. Add the vanilla extract at the end.
2. Line a small square or rectangular glass container with parchment paper. Press the batter down thoroughly with a large spoon. Freeze for 30 minutes.
3. Pull out and place on a wooden cutting board. Cut to desired bite sizes and serve. Keep refrigerated.

Tips and Variations:

1. It is essential that the seeds or nuts don't get burnt. Watch them closely as each oven differs a little. Pay special attention while toasting flax seeds as they are not good if scorched/burnt.

Date–Fig Balls (Orange–Lemon Flavour)

Naturally fibre-rich and sweet foods such as dates and figs, together with slow-burning nuts are a great snack for pick-up energy.

Ingredients:

10 dates (about ½ cup), pitted and cut small
10 figs, cut small
¼ cup unsalted toasted almonds (toast at 175°C for 8–10 minutes)
3–5 drops orange extract, or to taste (taste may vary depending on the brand)
1 tsp lemon juice
½ tsp lemon zest
A pinch of sea salt

Method:

1. Grind the dates, figs and almonds to a smooth, thick paste without water. Pulse and release often, and don't grind continuously.
2. Add the other ingredients and mix well.
3. Roll into little balls and serve. Keep refrigerated in an airtight container.

Date–Fig Balls (with desiccated coconut)

Ingredients:

10 dates (about ½ cup), pitted and cut small
10 figs, cut small
¼ cup unsalted toasted almonds (toast at 175°C for 8–10 minutes)
A pinch of sea salt
Desiccated coconut

Method:

1. Grind the ingredients to a smooth, thick paste without water. Pulse and release often, and don't grind continuously.
2. Roll into little balls and roll on a plate layered with desiccated coconut. Keep refrigerated in an airtight container.

Sweet Potato–Pumpkin Halwa

This is an excellent dish for asthmatics who are underweight.

Ingredients:

3 cups sweet potatoes or any sweet yam of your choice, cut into cubes, boiled and mashed
2 cups pumpkin or butternut squash, peeled and cut into cubes, boiled and mashed
4–5 tbsp powdered jaggery, or to taste
2 tbsp organic ghee or 1 tbsp tahini
A pinch of salt

Method:

1. Heat the mashed potatoes in a heavy-based stainless steel pan and add ghee or tahini and jaggery to taste. Serve warm or slightly chilled.

Oatmeal Cookies

Baked foods are normally not recommended for asthmatics, but this recipe is designed for those who cannot resist cookies once in a while. Be careful to use sparingly and in moderation.

Ingredients:

½ cup rice flour
½ cup rolled oats
¼ cup rice bran or organic coconut oil
¼ cup powdered jaggery
2 tbsp flax seeds
1 tbsp sunflower seeds
½ tsp vanilla extract
1/8 tsp sea salt
½ tsp baking powder
¼ cup de-seeded dates, cut small
1 tbsp unsweetened almond butter
3 tbsp unsweetened almond or any other non-dairy milk

Method:

1. Preheat the oven to 175°C or 400°F and bake for about 8–10 minutes or until lightly browned and cooked.

Tips and Variations:

1. Cool before serving.

Minty Vegan Home-made Chocolate

This recipe makes 5–6 pieces.

Chocolate should ideally not be consumed during the healing phase. But I added this recipe here for when your condition and immunity improves. Even then, this should be consumed in moderation (a small piece, not more than twice a month). This recipe is here for after you have followed the menu plan, home remedies and other recipes in this book for about 8–12 months.

Ingredients:

3 tbsp organic cold-pressed coconut oil
¼ cup organic raw cacao (I would recommend Mason & Co. or Earth Loaf)
2 tbsp coconut sugar
½ tsp maple syrup (optional, if you want it less bitter)
2 tbsp unsweetened smooth almond butter
2–6 drops of mint extract (start with two and add more as per taste and requirement)
A pinch of sea salt
¼ cup toasted almonds (toasted at 175°C for 8–10 minutes)
1-2 tbsp toasted sunflower seeds (toasted at 175°C for 12–15 minutes)

Method:

1. Melt the coconut oil and pour into a glass bowl.
2. Gradually stir in all the ingredients and whisk well.
3. In a silicone mould or paper cupcake moulds, place 3–4 toasted almonds and ¼ tsp toasted sunflower seeds at the bottom. Pour the chocolate on top and freeze for about 30–40 minutes.
4. Since this is an easy recipe you can make at home without using a thermometer and cacao butter, the chocolate melts easily, so keep it in the freezer.

Banana Bread

A delicious vegan banana bread recipe. Use this occasionally and in moderation after the healing phase.

Wet Ingredients:

1 cup mashed bananas
2 tbsp ground flax seeds
1/3 cup almond milk
1/3 cup coconut oil, melted, and a little more for oiling the pan
¼ cup high-grade pure maple syrup (do not use pancake syrup)
2 tsp organic vanilla extract

Dry Ingredients:

¼–1/3 cup organic coconut sugar
½ cup rolled oats
1¼ tsp aluminium-free baking soda
2 tsp aluminium-free baking powder
½ tsp sea salt
1½ cup barley flour
½ cup walnuts

Method:

1. Preheat the oven to 350°F or 190°C.
2. Oil the loaf or cake pan with a little coconut oil. Dust it with a little barley flour.
3. Mix the wet ingredients and slowly add the sifted dry ingredients, except the walnuts.

4. Pour the well-mixed batter into the loaf or cake pan. Sprinkle the walnuts on top.
5. Bake for 50–55 minutes or until a toothpick comes out clear.
6. Let it cool. Cut and serve along with your choice of sugar-free herbal tea. Herbal and non-milky teas help digest meals and desserts.

Tips and Variations:

You may add 2–4 drops of organic extract and 2 tsp of orange zest to this recipe for an added flavour. Do not use vanilla essence. Use good-quality vanilla extract or make it from vanilla beans.

23

Menu Planning

A lot of things need to be taken into consideration for anyone aiming to eat healthier. Some of these are:

1. Eating the right foods and avoiding harmful products such as commercial breads, refined sugar, commercial and most dairy products, poor-quality oils, etc.
2. Making food with better-quality ingredients.
3. Eating the right quantity as overeating can lead to acidity and sluggishness.
4. Not eating the right combination of foods. For example, fruits should not be mixed with beans and grains as that may lead to digestive discomfort or flatulence.
5. Not eating wholegrains with sweeteners as this promotes stagnation in the gut. Since the large intestine is a sister organ for the lungs, this directly impacts the lung function and repair.
6. Choosing to eat at the same time every day.
7. Choosing to eat food that is seasonally balanced. For example, you should have more of refreshing foods,

lemon, salads and raw salads in the summer, and long-cooked dishes and stews and soups in the winter.

8. Eating enough fermented foods on a daily basis.
9. Having digestion-friendly drinks each day.
10. Cooking well. For example, do not burn the oil in the pan, or under or overcook dishes. Opt for a variety of cooking styles.
11. Plan your menu. This makes all of the above more effective.

Menu Planning

Menu planning is an essential practice when it comes to working on your health. When doing so, always keep the following in mind.

1. Every meal must include a wholegrain or a cracked grain or a good-quality grain product.
2. Since grains are the centre of each plate, these must be of high quality. For example, if you are having chapatti for one meal in the day, every day, then make sure the flours used are pure and organic.
3. Don't have too many flour-based meals for several days in a row as this may make the system sluggish for lack of fibre.
4. Every meal must include at least one or two vegetables dishes. Vegetables added to fried rice or noodles do not qualify for the same. There must be separate vegetable dishes per meal.
5. Cook vegetables in a variety of ways. Having a subzi every day for every meal is nice but not balanced. There must be enough variety in the way you cook vegetables. This can include stir-fried dishes, salads, blanched and steamed

vegetables, matchstick vegetable dishes and long-cooked dishes.

6. Eat a lot of salads and sprouts. There are many dressings and dips in this book to encourage you to have salads.

7. Eat mineral-rich and refreshing dips and chutneys such as curry leaf–sesame or coriander–mint chutney, etc.

8. Each meal should have a high-quality, plant-based home-made protein dish. Occasionally, add a small quantity of high-quality, preferably organic animal protein, as and if desired.

9. Don't put oil in every dish on the plate. Make at least 1–2 dishes oil-free per meal.

10. Adding soups to meals makes them more nourishing. During the winter, have a soup almost every day while in the summer you can cut it down to a few times a week. Some people complain that it's too hot to have soup in the summer, but if hot dal works for us, why not soup?

11. Try to include some fermented food in every meal.

12. Keep most meals wholesome and nourishing as stated above. Once or twice a week you can opt for a one-bowl meal to give your digestive system a rest.

13. Keep one day in a week for lighter and oil-free cooking. Bring this up to two days in the week if you feel this works for you.

14. Dessert or snacks made with sweeteners should be had not more than twice a week, that too in moderation.

15. Do not overeat. Eating small quantities of each dish below is imperative. Overeating will not allow your body to receive healing energy from what you eat. Most recipes in this book serve 2–4 persons. If you live alone, you will need to adjust the quantity of the ingredients and maybe repeat a few dishes as leftovers every now and then.

Sample Spring/Summer menu

Week 1	Early morning	Breakfast	Mid-morning	Lunch	Evening drink or snack	Dinner
Suggested Time	Within half hour of waking up	7.30–9 a.m.	11–11.30 a.m.	12.30–1.30 p.m.	4–5 p.m.	Around 7 p.m.
Monday	½ tsp black seed oil with a few drops of organic raw honey + 6 soaked and peeled almonds + 1 soaked walnut + 1 cup cinnamon–clove tea	1 bowl of soft breakfast barley + 1 tsp toasted tan sesame seeds as garnish + Curry leaf–sesame chutney Blanched bok choy/ Amaranth greens	1 tbsp of home-made sunflower seeds trail mix + 1 small shot of freshly prepared amla juice	Boiled brown rice + Yellow moong dal + Pumpkin subzi 1/3 raw cucumber, sliced + 1 small piece oil-free lemon pickle	Brown rice tikkis with home-made chutney	1–2 besan leek chila or 1–2 chapatti + Lauki subzi + Mixed bean salad + side of steamed broccoli and beans with a dash of lemon juice or a drizzle of tahini lemon dressing

Week 1	Early morning	Breakfast	Mid-morning	Lunch	Evening drink or snack	Dinner
Suggested Time	Within half hour of waking up	7.30–9 a.m.	11–11.30 a.m.	12.30–1.30 p.m.	4–5 p.m.	Around 7 p.m.
Tuesday	5–6 raw tulsi leaves + 6 soaked and peeled almonds + 1 soaked walnut + 1 cup coriander seed tea	Red rice poha + 1 tsp toasted sunflower seeds and ½ tsp toasted flax seeds + Coriander–mint chutney + Blanched Chinese cabbage or cabbage	1 tbsp home-made sunflower seeds trail mix + 1 small shot of freshly prepared amla juice	1–2 wheat-free chapattis + Green moong dal + Bottle gourd subzi + Sprout salad	1 small bowl of roasted lotus seeds (Makhane)	Millet and vegetable patties (make extra for breakfast but pan-fry fresh in the morning. Keep uncooked patties in the refrigerator) + Basil or plain hummus + Raw salad

Week 1	Early morning	Breakfast	Mid-morning	Lunch	Evening drink or snack	Dinner
Suggested Time	Within half hour of waking up	7.30–9 a.m.	11–11.30 a.m.	12.30–1.30 p.m.	4–5 p.m.	Around 7 p.m.
Wednesday	½ tsp black seed oil with a few drops of organic raw honey + 6 soaked and peeled almonds + 1 soaked walnut + 1 cup cinnamon–clove tea	Leftover millet and vegetable patties + 1 small bowl blanched vegetable (for example, bok choy, broccoli, green beans) + Coriander-mint chutney	Sprout salad + 1 small shot of freshly prepared amla juice	2–3 red rice idlis + Vegetable sambar + Bitter gourd subzi + Mixed sprout salad + 1 tsp turmeric pickle	Steamed vegetable sticks with basil or plain hummus	1–2 besan–leek chila + Moth dal or leftover hummus + 1 small piece of broiled or steamed white-meat fish (optional) + Round gourd subzi (Tinda) + steamed vegetables with lemon flax dressing

Week 1	Early morning	Breakfast	Mid-morning	Lunch	Evening drink or snack	Dinner
Suggested Time	Within half hour of waking up	7.30–9 a.m.	11–11.30 a.m.	12.30–1.30 p.m.	4–5 p.m.	Around 7 p.m.
Thursday	5–6 raw tulsi leaves + 6 soaked and peeled almonds + 1 soaked walnut 1 cup coriander seed tea	Leftover red rice idlis + Curry leaf–sesame seeds chutney, or peanut chutney + Blanched bok choy/Amaranth greens	1 tbsp of home-made sunflower seeds trail mix + 1 small shot of freshly prepared amla juice	1–2 chapattis + Sautéed leeks + Bottle/round gourd subzi + 1 tsp turmeric pickle	1 helping of a seasonal organic fruit	Lung-healing khichdi + Pumpkin subzi + Mixed sprouts salad

Week 1	Early morning	Breakfast	Mid-morning	Lunch	Evening drink or snack	Dinner
Suggested Time	Within half hour of waking up	7.30–9 a.m.	11–11.30 a.m.	12.30–1.30 p.m.	4–5 p.m.	Around 7 p.m.
Friday	½ tsp black seed oil with a few drops of organic raw honey + 6 soaked and peeled almonds + 1 soaked walnut + 1 cup cinnamon–clove tea	Brown rice congee + 1 tsp black sesame seeds or home-made black sesame seed salt, ½ tsp toasted flax seeds, 1 tsp toasted pumpkin seeds + Blanched Chinese cabbage	1 tbsp of home-made sunflower seeds trail mix + 1 small shot of freshly prepared amla juice	Boiled brown rice or lemon white rice + Whole urad lentil (kaali dal) + Gobhi subzi + 1 tsp haldi pickle	Brown rice tikkis with home-made tikkis	1–2 chapattis or quinoa + Fish in mustard–carom marinade, or green moong dal + Wholesome salad with home-made dressing of choice + 1 tsp sauerkraut

Week 1	Early morning	Breakfast	Mid-morning	Lunch	Evening drink or snack	Dinner
Suggested Time	Within half hour of waking up	7.30–9 a.m.	11–11.30 a.m.	12.30–1.30 p.m.	4–5 p.m.	Around 7 p.m.
Saturday	5–6 raw tulsi leaves + 6 soaked and peeled almonds + 1 soaked walnut 1 cup coriander seed tea	Quinoa lemon rice style + 1 tsp white or black sesame seed salt + coriander–mint chutney	Mixed sprout salad + Lemonade made with salt, mint, and ½ tsp organic jaggery (optional)	Boiled brown rice + Methi–chana dal + Pumpkin subzi + Raw cucumbers, lettuce, sprouts with a dash of lemon juice or organic apple cider vinegar + 1 tsp toasted sesame seeds or home-made sesame seed salt	1 small helping of a seasonal organic fruit or kanten	2 chapatis or leftover quinoa lemon rice style + Kala chana salad or Kala chana kebabs + Lettuce, broccoli and avocado salad with any home-made dressing of your choice

Week 1	Early morning	Breakfast	Mid-morning	Lunch	Evening drink or snack	Dinner
Suggested Time	Within half hour of waking up	7.30–9 a.m.	11–11.30 a.m.	12.30–1.30 p.m.	4–5 p.m.	Around 7 p.m.
Sunday	6 soaked and peeled almonds + 1 soaked walnut + A cup of high-quality chamomile or lavender or rooibos tea	Brown rice tikkis + A small bowl of steamed broccoli or spinach with a dash of fresh lemon juice or apple cider vinegar + Coriander–mint chutney	1 date–fig ball + Freshly prepared cucumber, mint, lemon drink	Pan-fried polenta + Stir-fried vegetables + Mixed bean salad + A side of raw zucchini and cucumber salad + 1 tsp haldi pickle	1 small bowl of puffed rice, flax amaranth snack or a small helping of seasonal organic fruit	Boiled brown rice or brown rice salad + Yellow moong dal + Sautéed leeks, bok choy and broccoli + side of sprout salad (2–3 tbsp)

Sample Fall/Winter menu

Week 1	Early morning	Breakfast	Mid-morning	Lunch	Evening drink or snack	Dinner
Monday	½ tsp black seed oil with a few drops of organic raw honey	Soft millet with sweet vegetables	1 cup lotus root tea (after 6–8 weeks of consuming lotus root tea, have either a tulsi–white tea mix or lemon–chamomile tea. You can add a few drops of lemon to high-quality chamomile tea)	Pressure-cooked brown rice stir fried with white radish tops/greens	1 small bowl of oil-less puffed rice, flax amaranth snack	Chickpea–leek soup
	+	+		+		+
	6 soaked and peeled almonds	1 tsp toasted sesame seed, 1 tsp toasted sunflower seeds		Mixed healing lentil		Millet and vegetable patties
	+	+		+		+
	2 soaked walnuts	Blanched bok choy/Amaranth greens		Carrot and sweet peas		Steamed bok choy, pumpkin, green beans with carrot dressing
	1 cup cinnamon–clove tea			+ ⅓ raw cucumber, sliced		+ 1 tsp sauerkraut
				Curry leaf–sesame seed chutney		

Week 1	Early morning	Breakfast	Mid-morning	Lunch	Evening drink or snack	Dinner
Tuesday	Tulsi leaves	Leftover millet and vegetable patties	1 cup tulsi–mint tea, or tulsi green tea, or Rooibos tea	Pressure-cooked brown rice	Steamed vegetable sticks with basil or plain hummus	Broccoli–cauliflower soup
	+					+
	6 soaked and peeled almonds	+		+		Fried brown rice with cumin, onions and vegetables of your choice
		Curry leaves pressure-cooked chutney		Black chickpea curry/kala chana		
	+			+		+
	2 soaked walnuts	+		Pumpkin subzi		Moth dal
	+	Blanched or quick sautéed mustard greens		+		+
	1 pitted date			1 tsp haldi pickle		Pan-fried lotus root
						+ side of raw salad
	Ginger-lemon tea					+
						1 tsp sauerkraut

Week 1	Early morning	Breakfast	Mid-morning	Lunch	Evening drink or snack	Dinner
Wednesday	½ tsp black seed oil with a few drops of organic honey + 6 soaked and peeled almonds + 1 soaked walnut 1 cup cinnamon–clove tea	Soft corn dalia + Steamed water spinach (kalmi saag)	1 cup lotus root tea	Black millet and chana dal khichdi with seasonal vegetables like mooli + Fenugreek potatoes (methi–aloo) + side of mixed sprout salad + 1 tsp haldi pickle	1 small bowl of roasted lotus seeds	Pumpkin–sweet potato soup + White lobia sautéed with cumin, onion, garlic, and carrots seasoned to taste (no tomatoes) + Small helping of fried brown rice + Steamed lotus root and broccoli with lemon flax dressing 1 tsp sauerkraut

Week 1	Early morning	Breakfast	Mid-morning	Lunch	Evening drink or snack	Dinner
Thursday	Tulsi leaves + 6 soaked and peeled almonds + 2 soaked walnuts + 1 pitted date Rooibos tea or coriander seed tea	1–2 methi paranthas + A small bowl of mixed sprouts (alfalfa and fenugreek sprouts)	1 cup tulsi–mint tea, or tulsi tea, or licorice tea	Red rice–millet idli + Vegetable sambar + Mooli–mooli patta subzi 1 tsp oil-free lemon pickle	1 small helping of a seasonal organic fruit, or a helping of kanten, or a small piece of the home-made granola bar	Barley soup + 1–2 methi roti or parantha + Pumpkin subzi + Boiled chickpea salad or sautéed chickpea with vegetables + 1 tsp sauerkraut

Week 1	Early morning	Breakfast	Mid-morning	Lunch	Evening drink or snack	Dinner
Friday	½ tsp black seed oil with a few drops of organic honey + 6 soaked and peeled almonds + 1 soaked walnut + 1 cup cinnamon–clove tea	Red rice idli or dosa from leftover batter + a small bowl of mixed sprouts (broccoli and fenugreek sprouts)	1 small glass of carrot, apple, amla juice	1–2 chapattis + Moth lentils + Sautéed amaranth greens/chaulai saag	Steamed vegetable sticks with basil or plain hummus	Spinach and sweet potato soup, buckwheat cheela or roti, bottle gourd sabzi, lemon pickle

Week 1	Early morning	Breakfast	Mid-morning	Lunch	Evening drink or snack	Dinner
Saturday	Tulsi leaves + 6 soaked and peeled almonds + 2 soaked walnuts + 1 pitted date Ginger–lemon tea	Brown rice congee + Blanched bok choy/amaranth greens	1 cup lotus root tea	Stir-fried soba with vegetables + Lettuce, broccoli and avocado salad	1 small helping of a seasonal organic fruit or kanten	Clear broth ginger–lemon soup + 1–2 besan or moong dal chila + Yellow moong dal + Sweet potato tikkis

Week 1	Early morning	Breakfast	Mid-morning	Lunch		Evening drink or snack	Dinner
Sunday	Tulsi leaves	Besan toast made with un-yeasted sourdough bread	1 small glass of carrot, apple, amla juice	Bathua roti or parantha or brown rice stir fry with mooli pattas		Sweet potato tikkis with home-made chutney of choice	White rice or quinoa
	+						+
	6 soaked and peeled almonds	Coriander mint or curry leaf–sesame chutney					Fish in mustard–carom marinade or broiled fish with lemon
	+	Side of steamed Chinese cabbage and green beans		Mixed healing lentils or kulath ki dal			+
	2 soaked walnuts						2 tbsp grated mooli with lemon juice
	+						+
	1 pitted date			Turnip subzi			Lettuce and sweet potato salad
	+			+			+
	1 cup coriander seed tea			⅓ raw cucumber, sliced			1 tsp haldi pickle

24

International Recipes

There are many dishes from around the globe that are beneficial for healing asthma and other lung-related diseases. This section is for people who live outside India and whose local food may differ from people living in India. They can always follow some of the recipes from the previous chapters and choose from here.

I wrote this book sitting in India, but this section has many recipes that I tried myself and many others that are contributions from teachers, classmates from the Kushi Institute and friends from the macrobiotic community abroad. This section has some amazing healing recipes from friends from all over the world! I hope you enjoy it.

1. Miso Soup with White Radish Leek Soup with Ginger (page 243)
2. Grated Daikon Soup with Watercress (page 245)
3. Silky Carrot Soup with Orange (page 246)
4. Roasted Corn Miso Soup (page 248)
5. Quinoa and Millet Breakfast Porridge (page 250)
6. Kasha (page 252)

Miso Soup with White Radish

Miso is a naturally fermented probiotic food which cleanses the gut and helps rejuvenate the cells. It also pulls out radiation from the body and alkalizes the blood. It is one of the most healing soups. And it's simple. You can make it in just 7–10 minutes.

Ingredients:

½ cup onion, cut into half moons
½ tsp cold-pressed or toasted sesame oil

¾ cup leeks, cut half lengthwise, wash well and then cut thin diagonally

½ cup white radish, cut into thin half-moons

1½ tsp freshly grated ginger juice

1 thin spring onion, cut very fine for garnishing

½ tsp wakame flakes, soaked for 10 minutes

2½ tsp organic sweet white or organic yellow miso (buy organic, high-quality miso and not the commercial Japanese misos available as they often have MSG)

½ tsp organic barley or brown rice miso

1–1½ tbsp scallions or chives, cut fine for garnishing

Method:

1. In a stainless steel pot, heat the oil on a medium–low flame. Add the onions and a very tiny pinch of sea salt. Sauté for 2–3 minutes.

2. Add 3 cups of water, wakame along with the soaking water and bring to a gentle boil. Add the radish and after 1–2 minutes, add the leeks. Turn off the flame and stir in the miso.

3. Squeeze juice from the grated ginger into the soup. Pour the soup into serving bowls, garnish with scallions or chives and serve hot.

Tips and Variations:

1. Miso should not be reheated. So if you are making extra and wish to use it the next day, do not add the miso into the cooking pot. Add the miso to the soup you serve and put away the rest of the soup in the refrigerator. Add fresh miso later when you re-heat the soup.

2. You can add some noodles into the soup.
3. You can also add shiitake mushrooms into the soup. If using dried mushrooms, soak for 6–8 hours, discard the stems and slice thin. Shiitake mushrooms will need at least 25–35 minutes cooking with the onions and 2–3 more cups of water. The quantity of miso and ginger will also have to be re-adjusted slightly.
4. As the size of teaspoons and tablespoons varies across countries, I would recommend trying the soup before serving it. It should be moderately salty.
5. Miso soup can be made with any vegetables. The miso is usually 1 tsp per cup of grain. Darker misos are more hearty while yellow and white misos are sweeter and more delicious (easier for beginners).

Grated Daikon Soup with Watercress

This recipe has been contributed by Bettina Zumdick, a teacher, counsellor, author and humanitarian, and the founder of the Culinary Medicine School. It is taken from Zumdick's book *Authentic Foods*. This recipe is excellent for healing asthma and is very delicious. The grated daikon helps dissolve excess mucus in the lungs and airways, the shiitake mushrooms help open up the airways and the kombu-sea vegetable along with the watercress (or other slightly pungent greens such as mustard greens) strengthen the lungs.

Ingredients:

2 cups daikon, washed and finely grated
4–5 cups water, including kombu and shiitake soaking water

2 or 3-inch strip of dry kombu, soaked
4–5 dried shiitake, soaked, stems removed and diced
2–4 teaspoons of salt or to taste
1 bunch watercress, sliced into 1-inch strips (or other greens such as mustard greens)
¼ cup scallions, finely sliced
4–5 pieces of mochi, pan-fried (optional)

Method:

1. Place the water, kombu and shiitake in a pot. Cover and bring to a boil. Reduce the flame to medium and simmer for 5–10 minutes.
2. Remove the kombu and set aside for use in other dishes. Cover and simmer the shiitake for another 5 minutes. Add the daikon and sea salt. Cover and simmer over a low flame for another 10 minutes. Add the watercress and simmer for another minute.
3. Place pan-fried mochi in serving bowls, then ladle the soup into bowls and garnish with sliced scallions.

Silky Carrot Soup with Orange

This recipe is from Simone Parris, the founder and head chef at Simone's Kitchen in Antwerp. It serves 4–6 people.

This is a smooth, sweet soup with the delightful aroma of orange—adding 100 per cent natural organic essential oils to your cooking is like adding magic! As much as possible we only add essential oils to food after they have been removed from the heat.

Ingredients:

6 medium carrots, cut into thick diagonals

2 onions, diced
1 tbs extra-virgin olive oil
3 cm kombu
¼ cup rice flakes or oat meal
1 cup water
2 cups plain rice milk
Sea salt
2–3tbs soy cuisine (soy cream) (optional)
Ume vinegar
Zest of ½ orange
1 cup orange juice
2 drops of orange essential oil (optional but adds great flavour if you have it)

For Garnishing:

Fresh orange slices, ¼ cup fresh dill, parsley, chives or cilantro/coriander, washed, dried and finely chopped. You can also garnish with a drizzle of soy cream.

Method:

1. Heat a medium-sized soup pan. Add the olive oil and then sauté the onions with a pinch of sea salt.
2. Once the onions start smelling sweet and become translucent, add the carrots and another little pinch of sea salt. Sauté for a few more minutes.
3. Add the kombu and a cup of water, the rice milk and the rice flakes.
4. Bring to a boil and turn down to simmer for about 15–20 minutes or until the carrots are tender. Remove from heat.
5. Take out the kombu and add the zest, orange juice, essential oil, soy cream and 1 tbs of ume vinegar.

6. Using a hand-blender, puree the soup until smooth, adjusting the flavours as necessary.
7. Garnish and enjoy!

Tips and Variations:

1. Add 1 tsp fresh ginger (minced) to step 2.
2. Serve the leftover soup cold the following day.

Roasted Corn Miso Soup (with Wakame, Dried Shiitake, Pan-Fried Mugwort Mochi and Scallions)

This recipe is by Anna Aeschlimann, macrobiotic chef and educator. It is a summery, relaxing take on the classic miso soup. You can save it for when fresh corn is at its peak (frozen corn will not taste as good). Roasting the corn brings out its natural sweetness. Adding the mugwort mochi provides a chewy texture and a dramatic colour contrast.

Ingredients:

5 cups water, divided
2 small shiitake, soaked overnight
2 inches wakame, soaked in water
2 ears fresh sweet corn, still in their husks
2 tablespoons + ½ teaspoon chickpea miso
2 scallions, thinly sliced
3 pieces mugwort mochi, pan-fried
Safflower oil

To pan-fry the mochi:

1. Warm a plate in the oven at 200°F to place the mochi on.

2. Generously coat a cast-iron skillet with the oil and heat over medium–low heat.

3. Once the oil is simmering, add the mochi. Please note that most mochi is sold in vacuum-sealed packs of three. It is important to open the whole vacuum pack at once and use all three pieces as it will dry out very quickly once opened. Storing it for later use is not advisable.

4. Fry the mochi until golden brown, then flip it and brown the other side. You may need to add more oil.

5. Next, fry each edge of the mochi. Note that the edges will fry more quickly than the sides. You may need to hold the mochi in place with cooking chopsticks while frying the edges.

6. Once the edges are fried, place the mochi face-down again. Increase the heat to medium–high and pan-fry on the first side for 15 seconds. Flip the mochi and pan-fry the second side too. This last step prevents the mochi from collapsing once it is removed from the heat.

7. Remove the skillet from the heat. Place the mochi on a towel to drain the excess oil and then place it on the warmed plate. Please do not use a paper towel as it will stick to the mochi. It is important to warm the plate as this prevents the mochi from collapsing.

8. Allow the mochi to cool completely. Cut into small squares (1 piece of mochi will yield about eight croutons). It is important to let the mochi cool completely before cutting, otherwise it will lose its shape. Place six croutons in each soup bowl.

To make the soup:

1. Preheat the oven to 400°F. Place the corn (still in its husk) on a baking tray and roast for 30 minutes.

2. Remove from the oven. Allow it to cool before removing the husks and the silk. Cut the kernels off the cob (you should have about 1 cup). Place a bowl in your sink and scrape the 'milk' off the corn cobs into the bowl using a butter knife (this can get a bit messy, so doing it in the sink is helpful). The milk is the sweetest part of the corn, so don't skip this step!

3. Place ½ cup of the corn kernels and the corn milk in a blender with a cup of water. Blend on a high speed until completely smooth.

4. Remove the stems from the shiitakes and slice the caps thinly.

5. Remove the wakame from the water and cut into 1x1-inch pieces. Put the 4 cups of water, blended mixture, shiitakes, wakame, corn cobs and remaining corn kernels in a 2-quart soup pot and bring to a boil. Simmer for 30 minutes. Remove the cobs and shiitake stems and discard.

6. Place the chickpea miso in a suribachi and dilute with a ladleful of the soup. Add the diluted miso to the soup and simmer for 2 minutes (be careful not to let the soup boil after adding the miso as this would destroy the miso's enzymes). Add the scallions and simmer for a minute more. Taste and adjust the seasoning to your liking. Remember that this is meant to be a sweet, relaxing soup, not a salty one.

7. To serve, ladle the hot soup over the pan-fried mochi and serve immediately.

Quinoa and Millet Breakfast Porridge

This recipe serves 3–4 people.

Ingredients:

½ cup quinoa
½ cup millet
1 cup pumpkin, cut very fine
3½ cups water
A pinch of sea salt

Topping per person:

¾ tbs toasted sunflower seeds
1–2 tbs toasted pumpkin seeds
1 tbs toasted black or tan sesame seeds
3–4 toasted walnuts or almonds
¼ tsp shiso powder (optional)
¼ tsp nori flakes (optional)

Method:

1. Place all the ingredients in a stainless steel pot and bring
    to a boil. Lower the flame and place a flame tamer below
    the pot. Simmer for 20 minutes or till the grain is cooked
    and the water is absorbed.
2. Garnish and serve warm–hot.

Tips and Variations:

1. Quinoa millet for the main meals: You may omit the
    pumpkin and reduce the water to three cups and cook the
    same for lunch or dinner. It will be less porridge-like and
    will make for a delicious grain combination.

Kasha

This recipe by Susan L. Waxman, co-author of *The Complete Macrobiotic Diet* and co-director of SHI (Strengthening Health Institute), takes an hour to prepare. It serves four people.

This is a traditional Ukrainian recipe that is cooked in two parts. You can serve kasha as a grain dish or add it to bow-tie pasta for a delicious dish.

Ingredients:

1 cup roasted kasha
2 cups boiling water
1 pinch of sea salt (1/16–1/8 teaspoon)
1 cup of diced onion
1/2 cup of water
1/2–1 teaspoon olive oil
1/8 teaspoon sea salt

Method:

1. Place the roasted kasha in a pot.
2. In a separate pot, bring two cups of water to a boil. Add a small pinch of salt to the water and pour the boiling water over the kasha.
3. Cover the pot, reduce the flame and place a flame tamer under the pot.
4. Simmer on low heat for 20 minutes.
5. While the kasha is cooking prepare the sautéed onions.
6. Add a small amount of water to a skillet and add the diced onions. Begin to water sauté the onions. When the onions begin to change colour, add 1/16 teaspoon of salt and continue to sauté until the onions are translucent.

7. Add water as needed. When the onions are soft, allow the water to reduce and add ½–1 teaspoon of olive oil and another ¹⁄₁₆ teaspoon of salt. Use a wooden spoon to blend the salt, oil and onions and sauté for another 3–5 minutes.

8. When the kasha is cooked, place it in a serving dish. Add the sautéed onions and use a wooden spatula to mix the onions with the kasha.

Quinoa Salad with Walnuts, Grapes and Celery in a Lemon–Mustard Dressing

This recipe is from Carol Wasserman, a holistic nutritionist.

Ingredients:

1 cup red or tan quinoa, rinsed well
2 teaspoons mustard
Juice from 1 lemon (or use 2 tbs cider vinegar, brown rice vinegar, or red wine vinegar)
2 tablespoons extra virgin olive oil
¼ teaspoon sea salt, plus more to taste
½ cup halved grapes (or use ½ cup blueberries or dried cherries/cranberries)
½ cup walnuts, raw or dry roasted
1 stalk celery, chopped
¼ cup parsley, cilantro, mint, or basil chopped

Method:

1. Add the quinoa to a pot with 1½ cups of water and a pinch of sea salt. Bring to a boil. Cover, reduce heat and simmer for 15 minutes, or until all the water is absorbed.

2. Transfer cooked quinoa to a large bowl.
3. Add mustard, lemon juice, olive oil and sea salt to quinoa
    and stir to coat.
4. Taste and add more seasoning if needed.
5. Add the remaining ingredients and stir well.

Balsamic Brussels Sprouts

This recipe is by Masumi Goldman, yoga and meditation
teacher and a wellness advocate.

Ingredients:

1 lb (0.45 kg approx.) Brussels sprouts
1 tbs olive oil
2 tsp balsamic vinegar
¼ cup vegetable broth
⅓ cup crushed walnuts
salt and pepper (optional)

Method:

1. Cut the hard end off of each Brussels sprout and slice
    each one into fourths.
2. Heat 1 tablespoon of olive oil in a deep pan and sauté the
    Brussels sprouts for 5 minutes until they are golden in
    colour.
3. Add ¼ cup of vegetable broth and 2 teaspoons of balsamic
    vinegar to the pan. Stir the liquid and then cover the
    pan. Allow ingredients to simmer over a low flame for
    5 minutes.
4. Mix ⅓ cup of crushed walnuts into the pan. Add salt and
    pepper to taste.

Broiled Chilean Sea Bass

This recipe serves 4 people.

Ingredients:

Eight 3-ounce pieces of Chilean sea bass

Marinade:

3 tbs toasted sesame oil
1½–2 tbs high-grade maple syrup
1½ tbs tamari or organic shoyu
1 tbs mirin (optional)
About 1½ tbs lemon juice, or to taste
1 tbs fresh ginger juice
2–3 tbs fresh spring onions/scallions or chives as garnish

Method:

1. Whisk the marinade in a bowl. Marinate the fish for
   3–6 hours.
2. Broil the fish for 8–10 minutes or until done. The fish
   should be flaky soft and slightly crispy on the outside.
   Pull out and sprinkle the scallions 2–3 minutes.

Cucumber–Wakame Salad

This recipe serves 2–3 people.

Ingredients:

10 flakes wakame, crushed and soaked in 2–3 tbs water for
15 minutes

½ tsp maple syrup
½–1 tsp rice vinegar
½ tsp lemon juice, or to taste
½ tsp mirin (optional)
¼ tsp sea salt
1 tsp toasted sesame oil
½–¾ tbs organic or high-quality tamari
2½ cups cucumbers or 2–3 medium cucumbers, halved lengthwise and sliced thin

Method:

1. Rub ½ tsp salt into the cucumbers and press under a glass or ceramic plate with a heavy stone on it for two hours. Squeeze to remove the excess water.
2. Strain the water from the wakame.
3. Mix the maple syrup, rice vinegar, lemon juice, mirin, toasted sesame oil, tamari and cucumbers in a bowl. Add the wakame. Adjust seasoning to taste.

Pressed Salad, aka Quick Pickle

This recipe by Susan Ragsdale, a vegan macrobiotic chef and cooking teacher, serves 4 people.

Salting and pressing have the effect of cooking the vegetables. This fermentation makes the vegetables more digestible and preserves active enzymes, which are called probiotics. Any variety of cabbage may be used—green, red, Savoy or Napa (Chinese cabbage).

You will be massaging the ingredients with your hands, so use a large stainless steel or glass mixing bowl. Ensure that your hands are clean and free of soap. Also, be careful about tasting the pickle with your fingers and then putting your hands back in the bowl. Pickling promotes the growth of microorganisms and it's easy to introduce harmful bacteria that can make the pickle go bad. You can use the method described on page 192.

Ingredients:

Cabbage, cut into quarters. Use one quarter for this recipe. Remove the core. Thinly slice this quarter. You can use the stalk by cutting it into thin matchsticks.

Carrot, cut a small to medium-sized carrot

Cucumber, thinly sliced. If the skin is thick or the cucumber is waxed, peel it. If the seeds are large, they should be removed with a spoon before slicing. If using pickling cucumbers, slice them lengthwise into quarters, then into thin triangles.

Scallion, thinly sliced, or a finely grated quarter of a red onion with a ginger grater. You may also finely chop a small bunch of chives, the mildest form of onion.

¼ cup chopped fresh parsley

¼ teaspoon of salt

2 tsp umeboshi vinegar (If you don't have umeboshi vinegar, simply add an extra ½ teaspoon salt)

Sauerkraut (optional. I add a tablespoon to start the pickling process and add an interesting flavour)

½ cup roasted sunflower seeds (optional)

Method:

1. Ensure your hands are washed and free of soap.
2. In a large bowl, using both your hands, toss and massage these vegetables for a few minutes. The salt will lead to a liquid being released. Using a clean fork or chopsticks,

taste the salad. Do not put this utensil back into the salad for it will cause contamination. The salad should taste salty.

3. If you have a Japanese-style pickle press, transfer the vegetables into it and press. Use a glass or ceramic one, not plastic.

4. Otherwise, in the bowl, pat down the vegetables. Place a plate, with the right side up, on top of the vegetables. There should be at least ½ an inch of space between the edge of the plate and the bowl. This way, after the liquid is pressed out of the vegetables and the mound shrinks, the plate will not touch the sides of the bowl.

5. On top of the plate, place a 3–6 pound weight, such as a clean rock or another heavy object, such as a gallon jar filled with grains, beans or water.

6. The vegetables should be pressed for anywhere between half an hour to several hours. The longer the salad is pressed, the softer, sweeter and more interesting it becomes in flavour. If you have the vegetables in a pickle-press, you can put it into the refrigerator and keep overnight.

7. Once the salad is pressed, remove the plate and squeeze out the excess liquid with your hands. Put the pressed salad into a serving bowl. This liquid is called brine. Save it and keep it in the refrigerator. It can be in salad dressings in place of vinegar or lemon juice. It can also be splashed over vegetables for a tangy flavour boost or added to a dip.

Oil-free Radish Pickle

Eat 1–2 pieces of this pickle with meals to improve digestion. You can also refer to the section on pickles on page 191.

Ingredients:

4–5 cups white or red radishes, cut in half- or quarter-moons

Pickling liquid:

½ cup umeboshi vinegar
2¼ cups of water

Method: see page 192

Blanched Kale and Vegetable Salad with Gingered Carrot Pumpkin Seed Dressing

This recipe is by Amber Maisano, a macrobiotic chef, counsellor and teacher. This dish is bright, light, cleansing, cooked but crunchy, watery and hydrating. While each ingredient was chosen to support healing from asthma, the recipe is flexible. Feel free to adjust the amounts of the vegetables according to your preference.

It serves 8–10 people.

Ingredients (for dressing):

4 small orange carrots, sliced ⅛ of an inch diagonally
1¼ cup hot cooking water
2½ teaspoons fresh ginger juice
3 scallions, sliced in half horizontally
½ cup toasted pumpkin seeds, plus some for garnish
1 tablespoon and 1 teaspoon umeboshi vinegar

Ingredients (for salad):

2 cups cauliflower florets
1½ cups baby bok choy, sliced into 1-inch pieces

6 cups loosely packed curly kale, removed from stem and torn into large bite-sized pieces
3 stalks celery, sliced ⅛-inch diagonally
3 cups broccoli florets
1 bunch red radish, sliced into wedges
Splash of umeboshi vinegar, or ¼ teaspoon

Method:

To prepare the dressing:

1. In a large pot that is covered, bring 12 cups of water to a boil. Get a colander and skimmer, and place a bowl underneath the colander to catch draining water from blanched vegetables.
2. Once the water is boiling, submerge the carrots. After 5 seconds, remove them with a skimmer and transfer them to the colander. Place the carrots in the blender with the water and add the ginger juice. Add the remaining ingredients and blend until smooth.
3. Pour into serving dish and garnish with pumpkin seeds if desired.

To prepare the salad (for best results please read all the instructions first):

1. Bring the water to full boil again. Blanch each vegetable individually in the order they appear above, beginning with cauliflower. After the broccoli and before the red radish, you may add a splash of umeboshi vinegar to keep the radish looking bright.
2. To blanch, submerge the vegetables in the boiling water. Remove promptly with the skimmer and transfer to the

colander when they are bright in colour and you can faintly smell their aroma (be careful of the steam). Do not finish with a cold water bath.

3. The vegetables should be crisp but tender, and will vary in the amount of time needed for cooking. Additionally, you may prefer them cooked for slightly longer or shorter depending on the season and your condition. Feel free to adjust the cooking time according to your preferences, listening to the needs of your body. Given that, here is a guide for approximate cooking times.

- Cauliflower: 30 seconds to 1 minute
- Baby bok choy: 5 seconds (for more crunchy) to 30 seconds (for more sweet)
- Curly kale: 1 to 1½ minutes
- Celery: 1 minute
- Broccoli: 10 to 20 seconds
- Red Radish: Submerge completely then remove immediately, for brightest colour

4. Toss together or serve sectioned, with dressing.

Farro with White Beans and Kale

This recipe is by Susan L. Waxman. It has been taken from Waxman's book and serves 2–4 people.

Ingredients:

1 cup farro
2 cups water
1 cup diced onions
1 cup pre-cooked white beans

½ cup finely chopped kale
¼ cup extra virgin olive oil
¾ to 1 teaspoon sea salt
Sliced or whole garlic cloves, optional
Black or red pepper flakes, optional

Method:

1. Place the farro and water in a pot and bring to a boil.
2. Add a small pinch of sea salt.
3. Cover, place a flame deflector under the pot, and simmer on low heat for 35–40 minutes.
4. Pour enough olive oil into a separate pan to coat the bottom. Turn on the flame and begin to heat the oil.
5. Add the onions and sauté.
6. Add a few tablespoons water, ⅛ teaspoon sea salt and continue to sauté. Add the garlic and/or red pepper flakes now if you are using them.
7. Add the white beans and a little of the bean juice.
8. Add additional sea salt and continue to simmer over a medium–low flame for 10 minutes.
9. Add the chopped kale, fold to blend all of the ingredients together. Simmer for another 7–10 minutes.
10. Use a wooden utensil and add the farro to the vegetables and beans. Gently fold to blend the ingredients.
11. For additional richness and flavour, drizzle a little olive oil over the grain and add another small pinch of sea salt, about ⅛ of a teaspoon. Add black pepper if using.
12. Fold to blend all of the ingredients.
13. Place the farro in a serving bowl and cover with a bamboo mat until ready to serve.

Dandelion Tofu

This recipe is by Alexander Garberg, a macrobiotic cook.

Ingredients:

1 medium/large yellow onion
½–1 bunch dandelion greens
1 block tofu
2 tbs chickpea miso diluted in a little water
2 tsp mirin
¼ tsp oregano
¼ tsp black pepper
1 tsp sesame oil
¼ tsp toasted sesame oil
¼ tsp sea salt
Onion, sliced into thin half- or quarter-moons.

Method:

1. Heat a pan and add the sesame oil.
2. Add the sliced onion.
3. After a few minutes of sautéing, add a pinch of sea salt.
4. After a few more minutes of sautéing, add the finely chopped dandelion greens.
5. Crumble the block of tofu directly into the pan.
6. Add the mirin, oregano, black pepper, and rest of the sea salt.
7. Stir and cover for a few minutes.
8. Remove lid and add diluted chickpea miso.
9. Stir and let simmer for another minute.
10. Remove from heat and add toasted sesame oil.
11. Garnish with carrot flowers or finely cut scallion or chive.

Lentil and Quinoa-Stuffed Squash

This recipe is by Susan Beram.

Ingredients:

1 chopped onion
¼ chopped garlic
1½ chopped kale
1½ shredded carrots
1 shredded broccoli
1 shredded cabbage
1 cup brown lentils
1 cup quinoa
Thyme
Pepper
Cumin
Some chopped almonds
Some currants
6 acorn squash

Method:

1. Steam the onions, garlic, kale, carrots, broccoli and cabbage. Allow to cool.
2. Cook 1 cup brown lentils in 3 cups of vegetable stock or water. Take 1 cup quinoa, rinsed and cooked in 1½ cup vegetable stock or water, covered for 20 minutes.
3. Combine the cooked lentils, quinoa and the steamed vegetables with the thyme, pepper, cumin, chopped almonds and currants.
4. Cut, prick back and cook six acorn squash face down at 350 degrees in a baking pan for 45 minutes to an hour.

Check with a fork to see when they are done. They should be firm and soft. When the squash is done, stuff it with lentils, vegetables and the quinoa mixture.

Kezia's Mustard Dressing

This recipe is by Kezia Snyder, a natural foods cook and teacher. This dressing can go over steamed or blanched veggies or a raw salad. It is simple and delicious and adds a wonderful flavour to any basic preparation. You can vary it as you like, with the addition of different herbs such as oregano, thyme, parsley or dill.

Depending on the amount of vegetables you want to coat with this dressing, you may need to increase the quantity of the ingredients used. This recipe makes enough dressing for two generous servings of vegetables. For optimum healing benefits, all the ingredients should be organic and local as far as possible.

This dressing is especially delicious over cooked broccoli. Mustard is known to be particularly good for health in combination with cruciferous vegetables.

Ingredients:

2 tbs olive oil
1 tbs grainy mustard
1 small clove of pressed garlic (you can also use a small amount of minced scallions, or chives, or onion or shallots)
A few drops of umesu (plum vinegar) and apple cider vinegar, to taste
A very small amount of water or vegetable broth, to desired consistency.

Method:

1. Mix all ingredients well.
2. Taste for degree of saltiness, it should be slightly more than what you would like, as it will soak in and disperse over the vegetables.

Japanese Carrot–Ginger Dressing

This recipe is by Carol Wasserman, a holistic nutritionist.

Ingredients:

1 cup grated carrots
1 tsp mustard
1 tbs chopped onion
2 tsp minced fresh ginger root
1 tbs soy sauce
1 tbs brown rice vinegar
2 tbs extra virgin olive oil (or sesame oil)
1 tsp agave nectar or honey (optional)
2 or 3 tablespoons water, or more as needed to facilitate blending

Method:

Add all ingredients to a blender or food processor. Blend until creamy.

Orange Flax Dressing

This recipe serves 2–3 people.

Ingredients:

2 tbs organic cold-pressed flax seed oil or olive oil
½ tsp maple syrup, or raw honey, or 1 tsp unflavoured brown rice syrup/nectar
½ tsp rice vinegar
1½–2 tsp umeboshi vinegar, or to taste
2 tsp fresh lemon juice
2 tbs fresh orange or kinnow juice (optional)
1 clove of garlic, crushed/pressed
A generous pinch of black pepper

Method:

1. Place in a jar and shake well. Serve over salads or steamed or blanched vegetables of your choice.

Pumpkin Seed Dressing

This recipe serves 2–4 people. This depends on whether you are using it as a side salad or with a main salad.

Ingredients:

1 cup pumpkin seeds
1½ tsp umeboshi paste
1 tsp lemon juice
2 cups fresh flat leaf parsley (I prefer a lot of parsley)

Method:

1. Blend all ingredients in a food processor to a creamy smooth consistency.

Sweet Potato Kabocha Mash

This recipe serves 2–3 people.

Ingredients:

1 cup kabocha pumpkin or butternut squash, cut into cubes
2 cups sweet potatoes or Japanese yam, peeled and cut into cubes
A pinch of sea salt
½ tsp umeboshi paste
1 tbs and 1 tsp tahini

Method:

1. Bring the vegetables with a cup of water and a generous pinch of salt to a boil. Simmer for 10–12 minutes or until they are soft. Turn off the flame and let this cool.
2. Blend to a creamy, thick texture. Add the tahini and umeboshi paste and add salt to taste. Serve at room temperature.

Tips and Variations:

1. The above recipe is inspired by macrobiotic counsellor and educator Warren Kramer. I cooked under his guidance for his patients and tried something similar then. This recipe has some changes from the original.
2. You can add a dash of lemon juice for a summery flavour.

Dessert Salad

This recipe is by Sylvia Ruth Gray, author of *Eating Animals: Would George Ohsawa and Michio Kushi Be Vegan Today?*

Ingredients:

Fresh beets (any colour) or fresh carrots (any colour)
Medium-sized lemon
Small onion
Raw garlic
Oil
Salt
Fresh basil or mint

Method:

1. Cook the beets or carrots in boiling water until tender. (It is easiest to peel beets after cooking and easiest to scrub or peel carrots before cooking.)
2. Finely chop the onion, combine with ¼ tsp salt and let it sit.
3. Remove blemishes from lemon peel and slice crosswise into ¼-inch slices. Carefully remove seeds. Place lemon slices, peeled garlic cloves, ¼ tsp salt and 2 teaspoon oil in a food processor and pulverize.
4. Dice cooked beets (or slice cooked carrots) and toss with the onion–salt and lemon–garlic–oil mixture. Allow 24–48 hours before serving.
5. Toss with finely cut basil or mint at serving time.

Almond Arame Dish

This recipe serves 3–4 people.

Ingredients:

2 onions, cut into half-moons
3–4 carrots, cut into matchsticks

¼ tbs arame to taste
1½ tbs fresh ginger juice
½ tsp sea salt
Tamari or shoyu to taste (keep the salt low as this dish is sweet and creamy)
¼ cup fresh spring onions/scallion or chives as garnishing
1 tbs cold-pressed sesame oil
2 tbsp unsweetened pure, smooth almond butter

Method:

1. Rinse and soak the arame in enough water to cover it. Let it soften for about 30–40 minutes.
2. Sauté the onions in a stainless steel or ceramic pan. Cover the bottom of the pan with the onions and add a little water enough to just about cover the onions.
3. Layer the carrots on top of the onions without disturbing or stirring the onions.
4. Layer the softened arame over the carrots without disturbing the onions and carrots.
5. Add half of the arame soaking water. This should just about cover the onions and part of the carrots. Cover and simmer for about 20 minutes. Check to see the vegetables do not burn. Add a little water if needed.
6. Mix the almond butter with the remaining arame soaking water that will make the almond butter less sticky and a little softer and watery.
7. Add the ginger juice, a little tamari (about 1–2 tsp) and the almond butter. Stir well and simmer for 30–60 seconds. Turn off the heat and stir in the scallions. Serve hot.

Tips and Variations:

1. You can make the same dish without the almond butter and arame for a light, gingery version. You can add green beans or lotus root instead of the arame.

Cannelloni Beans with Dandelion Greens

This recipe is by Susan Beram.

Ingredients:

1 cup dry cannelloni beans
1 bunch dandelions
1–3-inch pieces of kombu
1 bay leaf
¼ teaspoon salt
1 tablespoon white miso
Garlic clove, chopped
Olive oil

Method:

1. Rinse the beans. Bring the water to a boil and pour over beans to cover. Soak overnight.
2. The next day, discard the soaking water. Cover the beans in a pot with water that goes an inch over the beans.
3. Add the kombu and bay leaf to the pot.
4. Bring to a light boil and remove the scum.
5. Simmer gently, pot uncovered, till the water is down to the level of the beans.
6. Add water to keep the level ½ an inch above the beans.

7. Continue to simmer until cooked. Add cold water when needed.

8. Once the beans are soft, dilute 1 tablespoon white miso in some water and add to beans with ¼ teaspoon salt.

9. Add chopped garlic clove.

10. Continue cooking for twenty minutes.

11. Add the dandelions (see directions below) and serve.

Prepping Directions for the Dandelions:

1. Remove inner core, which is bitter, and cut the rest into slices.

2. Wash to remove all grit.

3. Bring water to a boil with no salt.

4. Boil dandelions for 3–5 minutes till sweet and drain.

5. Saute quickly in olive oil, with a pinch of sea salt.

6. Add to beans and serve.

Sample Menu Plan

Week 1	Early morning	Breakfast	Mid-morning	Lunch	Evening drink or Snack	Dinner
Monday	⅓–½ tsp cold-pressed coconut oil with a drop of doTerra oregano oil	Quinoa and millet porridge	(optional)	Boiled brown rice	Mixed sprout salad with a drizzle of your choice of dressing	Broccoli–cauliflower soup
		+ 1 tsp toasted sesame seeds or home-made sesame seed salt, ½ tsp toasted sunflower seeds, 1 tsp roasted pumpkin seeds		French lentils		+
	6 soaked and peeled almonds			Bok choy and lotus root salad		Brown rice patties from leftover brown rice or fried brown rice
	+			Pressed salad, aka quick pickle		
	1–2 soaked walnuts	A side of steamed asparagus				Mixed bean salad
	1 cup cinnamon–clove tea					Matchstick vegetables
						1 tsp sauerkraut

Week 1	Early morning	Breakfast	Mid-morning	Lunch	Evening drink or Snack	Dinner
Tuesday	4–5 raw organic basil leaves or holy basil leaves (you could get a large pot)	Brown rice congee	A small bowl of puffed rice, flax and amaranth snack	Kasha	A small portion of seasonal organic mixed blue and black berries or poached apricots	Miso soup with onions, bok choy, white radish/daikon and broccoli
	6 soaked and peeled almonds	3–4 toasted walnuts, 1 tsp toasted pumpkin seeds, 1 tsp black sesame seed salt		Almond arame dish		Fried brown rice
	+	A bowl of mixed sprouts—broccoli sprouts, alfalfa sprouts, radish sprouts with a dash of lemon juice		Small bowl of pinto or fava beans		Leftover pinto or fava beans from lunch or a small piece of steamed or broiled fish or yellow moong lentils
	1–2 soaked walnuts			Blanched bok choy, green beans, broccoli sprouts, cucumbers and lettuce with pumpkin seed dressing		2 slices steamed kabocha or butternut squash or any summer squash
	1 cup cinnamon–clove tea					1 tsp sauerkraut

Week 1	Early morning	Breakfast	Mid-morning	Lunch	Evening drink or Snack	Dinner
Wednesday	½ tsp cold-pressed coconut oil with a drop of doTerra oregano oil	Soft barley breakfast	Ame kudzu	Quinoa/brown chickpeas or Farro and white bean salad	Steamed vegetable sticks with basil or plain hummus	Kabocha and Japanese yam soup
		Roasted almonds				Soba, rice or udon noodles
	6 soaked and peeled almonds	A bowl of mixed sprouts: broccoli sprouts, alfalfa sprouts, radish sprouts with a dash of lemon juice		Steamed kale, broccoli, bok choy, carrots, snap peas with Kezia's mustard dressing or leftover pumpkin seed dressing		Pan-fried tofu with stir-fried broccoli, lotus root, carrots, bok choy, cabbage and radish sprouts
	+					
	1–2 soaked walnuts					
	1 cup cinnamon–clove tea			1–2 pieces white radish ume pickle		1 tsp sauerkraut

Week 1	Early morning	Breakfast	Mid-morning	Lunch	Evening drink or Snack	Dinner
Thursday	4–5 raw organic basil leaves or holy basil leaves (you could get a large pot)	Soft millet with sweet vegetables or softly cooked broken corn (polenta)	A small bowl of puffed rice, flax and amaranth snack	Pan-fried tempeh Lettuce, broccoli and avocado salad	Apricot kanten	Watercress and grated daikon soup Aduki beans sautéed with onions, butternut, carrots
	6 soaked and peeled almonds +	1 tbs roasted pumpkin seeds, 1 tsp roasted sunflower seeds		1 tsp sauerkraut		Millet and vegetable patties
	1–2 soaked walnuts	Side of steamed bok choy				Pressed salad, aka quick pickle
	1 cup cinnamon-clove tea	+ home-made sweet vegetable jam				

Week 1	Early morning	Breakfast	Mid-morning	Lunch	Evening drink or Snack	Dinner
Friday	4–5 raw organic basil leaves or holy basil leaves (you could get a large pot) 6 soaked and peeled almonds + 1–2 soaked walnuts 1 cup cinnamon–clove tea	Leftover millet and vegetable patties With choice of home-made dip or chutney A bowl of mixed sprouts: broccoli sprouts, alfalfa sprouts, radish sprouts with a dash of lemon juice	A small bowl of puffed rice, flax and amaranth snack	Pressure-cooked brown rice Brown lentils, stir-fried vegetables with a dash of lemon juice or apple cider vinegar + Steamed radish greens or steamed bok choy and green beans	1–2 tbs sunflower seed trail mix	Yellow moong lentils or green moong lentil soup Brown rice Stir-fried vegetables of choice or matchstick vegetables 1 tsp sauerkraut

Week 1	Early morning	Breakfast	Mid-morning	Lunch	Evening drink or Snack	Dinner
Saturday	½ tsp cold-pressed coconut oil with a drop of doTerra oregano oil	1 slice of unyeasted sourdough bread with basil or lemon hummus	Ame kudzu	Millet mashed potatoes with herbed mushroom sauce	A small portion of seasonal organic mixed blue and black berries or poached apricots	Silky carrot soup
				+		+
	6 soaked and peeled almonds	Side of blanched kale				Quinoa salad with lemon–mustard dressing
	+			Sautéed or steamed leeks		Basil or lemon hummus, or a piece of broiled fish
	1–2 soaked walnuts			+		
				Black-eyed peas sautéed with cumin, turmeric, salt, garlic, onions.		+
	1 cup cinnamon–clove tea					A side of boiled broccoli, carrots and bok choy
				+		
				Pumpkin sweet potato mash		+
						Pressed salad aka, quick pickle
				1 tsp sauerkraut		

Week 1	Early morning	Breakfast	Mid-morning	Lunch	Evening drink or Snack	Dinner
Sunday	4–5 raw organic basil leaves or holy basil leaves (you could get a large pot) 6 soaked and peeled almonds + 1–2 soaked walnuts 1 cup cinnamon–clove tea	Softly cooked farro or brown rice (soaked the previous night in four times the water) + Blanched bok choy with radish microgreens	Carrot-apple juice	Red rice idlis Vegetable sambar or French lentils + Steamed kabocha, white radish and broccoli with Japanese carrot ginger dressing or a lemon–tahini dressing	A small bowl of leftover hummus and cucumbers	Creamy cauliflower soup Quinoa lentil loaf or quinoa lemon–rice style Quick sautéed carrots and kale Mixed sprouts salad

25

FAQs

This chapter lists out a few frequently asked questions about one's diet, conceptions and misconceptions about healthy eating.

Q. How is brown rice different from white rice?

A. Brown rice, also known as unpolished rice, is how nature gave us rice in its original form, with all the layers, fibre, nutrients and minerals intact. When you remove all the good layers, then the bulk of the rice—the starchy part— left behind is called white rice. Bulk in a grain adds bulk to the body and hence eating too much white rice may lead to weight gain. However, this does not happen with brown rice as the natural nutrients, minerals and fibre help metabolize the starchy part.

All wholegrains, especially brown rice, have abundant life force energy. When you sow one grain of rice, you get back a thousand grains. Hence it has a rejuvenating power and multiplies life energy. But if you sow white rice, you will get nothing back. Also, brown rice can be stored for hundreds of years without getting spoilt. This shows how much life force it carries.

Brown rice should be eaten regularly, while white rice should be consumed occasionally. If you ask me, brown rice should simply be called rice and white rice should be called polished and refined rice.

Q. Are rolled oats healthy?

A. Rolled oats are an average food in terms of nutrition and is a good option to use in desserts and granola bars, or when travelling with limited options available. However, steel-cut oats and whole oats offer deeper nourishment.

Q. Is dalia (cracked wheat) healthy?

A. We should consume the different types of grains in the following order:

1. Whole and unprocessed (most often)
2. Cracked grains (often)
3. Grain products (few times a week)
4. Commercial-quality grain products (rarely or if you have no choice)

Dalia is basically a cracked grain and can be used several times a week. However, those who have weak digestion must avoid wheat dalia and choose the barley, millet, corn or bajra versions. Soak dalia overnight to soften the grains and make them more digestible.

Q. My doctor has told me not to have too much wholegrain as its fibre is bad for me. He said I shouldn't have brown rice often. What do I do?

A. Brown rice is one of the most nourishing foods on the planet. It is both the seed and fruit. Most doctors find immediate, and sometimes only temporary, solutions to problems. They may or may not be aware of the natural and long-term solutions. They mean no harm but they simply may not know enough about the healing properties of natural and whole foods. That is because not every doctor has studied nutrition. In four years of their studies to become a doctor, they have less than twenty hours focused on nutrition. Recently, the number of doctors who are open to natural ways—called functional doctors—and are more aware about smart natural solutions to health problems has increased.

Some people are not able to absorb nutrients from brown rice due to poor eating habits that may have weakened their digestive system. To be able to absorb nutrients from brown rice, one needs to pay attention to the following factors:

1. Pay attention to the quality of brown rice used. Always use high-quality organic brown rice.
2. Soak brown rice for at least 8–12 hours. Soaking rice makes it more digestible.
3. Bring rice to one boil or pressure and then simmer for 45 minutes on a low flame to make it more digestible. Making it on a high flame or with less water and for a short time will not allow the rice to cook properly and hence will not allow you to receive the nutrition and energy it has to offer.

4. Learn about natural ways to improve your digestion rather than accepting that you won't ever have brown rice. If your digestion is weak, you should have brown rice 2–3 times a week only, that too cooked softly.

5. Develop awareness about the steps to help improve digestion. This depends on your body type and may require you to consult a macrobiotic counsellor to learn how to use brown rice.

6. Develop a long-term perspective. Brown rice is a very pure food that expels toxins from the body. If you have brown rice while continuing to consume sugar, processed foods and ice cream or other forms of dairy, then you may go through some digestive discomfort or pain. The key to allowing brown rice to nourish you is an intelligent and patient step-by-step action plan.

Q. What should I eat?

A. You should follow a simple format:

1. A small quantity of any of these grains: brown rice, foxtail millet, barnyard millet, jowar, barley, finger millet, buckwheat, white rice, pasta, rice noodles, etc.

2. A large quantity of one to two vegetable dishes.

3. A protein dish: beans, lentils, or a small quantity of choice of animal protein which is free of toxins and hormone injections.

4. Have fermented foods: a small piece of a digestive home-made oil-free pickle.

5. Include a soup often, especially pureed vegetable soups.

6. Include a salad often.

7. Include blanched or boiled vegetables with lemon juice or your choice of dressing at least at one meal per day.

Q. They say that we should have only local foods. Then why have quinoa which is not indigenous to my country?

A. I encourage the use of local grains along with a few extraordinarily healing foods that may not be local. This is keeping in mind the fastest and least troublesome way to heal.

It is not necessary to include quinoa in one's diet. It is often recommended during the healing phase for some people because it is easy to digest and assimilate. It has more complete forms of protein and is rich in magnesium as well. In fact, quinoa was worshipped by many civilizations, including the Aztecs who believed that it helped the human body heal and recover quickly, and also had spiritual reverence.

If the reason why you have fallen sick or gained weight is because of consuming foods such as pastas, pizzas, ice creams, processed cheese and restaurant food, then you should not be prejudiced against healthy foods that are not indigenous to your country. Not that you want to have this every day, but if you are sick and recovering from any disease, then it helps you heal faster. It's perfectly fine to stop using these once you feel you have gained strength and can easily digest heartier wholegrains.

Also, if you have had a lot of animal proteins in the past then your diet needs to be high in healthy plant-based proteins as well. Quinoa has many essential amino acids that are easy to digest and assimilate even if you have a weak digestion. Healthy plant-based protein and natural fat helps pull out toxic protein and fat buildup. In India, amaranth is a close cousin of quinoa and should be used often.

Q. What are xenoestrogens?

A. Estrogen is a human hormone. Xenoestrogens are chemical compounds that imitate estrogen.

In today's world there are many chemicals used in shampoos, perfumes, make-up, cleaning products and in processed and packaged food. Chemicals are also sprayed on our crops, vegetables and fruits. They also find their way in through bad-quality cookware and plastics used in our kitchen and restaurants. These chemicals are also found in poor-quality electronic gadgets. All these chemicals enter our body and mimic the hormones, disrupting the functioning of the endocrine system. Since most of these chemicals are not biodegradable, they get embedded into the fat cells of our body. This is one of the leading causes of many modern-day diseases, including cancer. In fact, these chemicals are said to be one of the leading causes for breast cancer. It is best to choose environment-friendly products for personal and planetary health.

Q. We are vegetarians and eat no dairy products and white sugar. Isn't this already balanced? Do we need to do anything else?

A. In this day and age, being merely vegetarians or eating primarily plant-based food is not enough. Our body requires nutrients and energy in a certain ratio from different cooking methods. Educating ourselves about our body type and making constant and active changes to our diet is necessary. One shouldn't eat anything in excess either. Eating too much grain or too much or too little salt, or too much oil or too much fruit is not healthy either. Health comes from eating everything in the right proportion.

Q. My child doesn't like to eat vegetables. What can I do?

A. This is a very common trend. There are three reasons for this. One is genetics and what the mother ate during pregnancy. The second is white and other simple sugars. If the child is eating too many simple sugars and desserts, then his or her palate is so sweetened, which does not allow him or her to enjoy the natural sweetness and taste of vegetables. The key to help them eat more vegetables is to reduce their intake of white sugar, refined flour and processed foods. The third reason is chemicals. If the child is consuming packaged foods such as chips, cookies, two-minute noodles or soups, then their palate is too stimulated by the chemicals in these foods to enjoy natural food. They have to go through a few months of detox before they are in a position to accept healthy food. You can initially use more seasoning and fat in meals during the transition period, if needed, and gradually move to healthier foods as the child's body and palate cleanses.

Q. Why is asthma called a cold disease?

A. The lungs are located in the upper part of the body. Extra mucus is also stored here. If that happens, it is a sign that the body has low circulation and that the energy is not flowing to the lower parts of the body easily. Besides circulation, the heat metabolism in the body too is affected.

In the case of people who get colds often, their lower body and lower chakras are less active and warm. This is why the body expels excess toxic buildup through the upper channels—the nose, chest and throat. Their abdomen and root chakra are not as strong and the lower organs of elimination are not functioning to their full capacity.

There is another more subtle mechanism in action. The abdomen is the lower centre of the body, as in many traditional systems, the heart is the middle or upper centre. There are many ways to classify the upper centres but the lower centre is always the hara, or the abdomen. If the lower centre, which is responsible for warm and deeper circulation, is weak, there is a disconnect between the lower and upper body, which leads to the body not functioning optimally.

Q. If I eat sugar and burn the extra calories in the gym, is that okay?

A. Eating food is not only about calories and nutrients. There are many other ways each food acts and reacts within the body. Some foods benefit the body while the others weaken the immune system.

Sugar is detrimental to the functioning of the whole body. It is not just that it is high in calories. Here are a few ways it impacts the body:

1. Bad bacteria feed on sugar in the gut. Hence, eating sugar promotes the increase of bad bacteria.
2. Sugar weakens the adrenal glands and reduces the daily energy available to us.
3. Sugar causes inflammation in the body, which is a precursor to many modern-day diseases.
4. Sugar creates instability in the blood sugar levels and weakens the pancreas, spleen and digestion. If the digestion is weak, one's nutrient assimilation is weak. This affects the immune function.
5. Sugar triggers acidity. A person with more acidic blood is more prone to allergic reactions.

Q. Are all fermented foods good for us?

A. Food fermented with salt and certain healthy starters such as sourdough starters or koji are healthy. Foods fermented without salt such as alcohol are not healthy. Salt in fermented foods creates the element of health.

Q. I take apple cider vinegar everyday in the morning. Is that okay?

A. Apple cider vinegar is a refreshing addition to salads and salad dressings weekly or occasionally, but it may not be so great when consumed as a health tonic on a daily basis. The quality is of utmost importance. Choose only organic and natural vinegars. Avoid synthetic vinegars, as they can be harmful to health.

Q. Should we use soaking water for rice and beans?

A. It is okay to use soaking water for grains. But water should be discarded for all beans, except dark beans, such as black soybeans, brown chickpeas (kala chana), red black-eyed peas and aduki beans. If your digestion is sensitive, discard the soaking water for grains.

Q. Beans do not suit me. They give me digestive discomfort and flatulence? What can I do?

A. The gut needs foods rich in fibre and fermented foods. If you have eaten foods that are not healthy for many years, and hence suffer from digestive problems, then they might find beans difficult to digest.

To make beans more digestible you may cook beans with 1-2 bay leaves and/or a small postage stamp-size piece of kombu. It is also advisable to have these cooked very soft and in small quantities.

Beans look like and nourish the kidneys. According to macrobiotics, kidneys are considered as the root of life. It's said that the spirit resides in the kidneys. If the kidneys are not properly nourished then one cannot reach their best health potential.

Q. I eat only raw food. Is that okay?

A. Raw foods are excellent and good to consume as part of a healthy regime. It is good to have more of such foods in the summer than during any other season.

However, only raw foods are not healthy as the body does not receive enough fire energy to support proper circulation and maintain a healthy heat metabolism. Sometimes consuming excessive raw foods can make a person weak and even lead to poor circulation and adrenal fatigue. Also, raw foods should be as organic as possible.

One man's medicine is another man's poison. This is very true for raw foods. It suits those who have more heat and a pitta dosha but can be detrimental for those with a vata dosha.

Q. If I give up milk and cheese, where will I get calcium from?

A. We get healthy calcium from beans, dark leafy greens, sea vegetables and algae (such as spirulina tablets or hijiki), almonds, sesame seeds, dates, figs, broccoli, amaranth and many other non-dairy foods. Trace amounts of calcium are found in almost all foods.

Calcium from dairy products are difficult for the body to absorb. These days, cows are injected with growth hormones so that they can produce more milk. Also, they are given antibiotics for hygiene and safety. All this enters the blood stream of human beings when they consume dairy products. Hence, dairy ends up being more acidic and harmful than helpful. Highly processed cheese like cheese slices and cream cheese are very often not cheese. They contain loads of oil and act like plastic in the body—it covers the cells and tissues and blocks blood circulation.

Q. I go to the gym and eat eggs every day. My instructor says that I need the protein to work out. Is this okay?
or
Eggs are healthy. What's wrong with eggs?

A. Eggs are considered to be yang/contractive foods according to macrobiotics. In fact, eggs are known to have more masculine energy than chicken. It is, after all, the energy of an entire chicken condensed into an egg.

Eggs are known to benefit the left brain, which may be why people who are very logical are called eggheads. Also, since eggs come from the reproductive system of an animal, they have a negative impact on the reproductive organs of human beings.

Eggs are not a healthy part of one's diet. If one chooses to consume eggs, they must limit the quantity. They are high in fat and protein content and offer instant energy which people enjoy. But too many eggs can lead a person to become angry or irritable.

We are at our best when we align ourselves with nature. In the morning, the sun rises and the day opens up. We must have foods that help us open up and expand. Hence traditional breakfast dishes include foods that are softer and have more water content such as porridge, dalia, poha, juice, fruits, etc. When we have eggs for breakfast, we go in the exact opposite direction. If we have eggs for breakfast, we start the day with strong, contractive energy that is the opposite of the sun's rising and expanding energy.

Q. Is a vegan diet healthy?

A. Please refer to Chapter 2.

Q. Is a vegetarian diet healthy?

A. Please refer to Chapter 2.

26

The Macrobiotic Viewpoint of Asthma

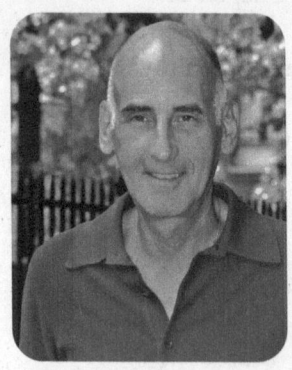

Denny Waxman, a macrobiotic counsellor and author of *The Complete Macrobiotic Diet* and founder of the Strengthening Health Institute (SHI), has helped thousands of clients recover their health using the macrobiotic diet and lifestyle. He can be contacted at dennywaxman@dennywaxman.com.

From my experience and understanding of macrobiotics, there is a natural, progressive development of illness. The first stage begins with physical and/or mental fatigue. The second stage includes aches, pains and stiffness. The third stage is blood-related disorders.

Essentially, fatigue signifies that our overall condition is becoming acidic. Aches, pains and stiffness signify that blood and lymph circulation are affected. In the third stage, blood quality is affected or compromised. The most common symptoms of this stage are allergies, skin diseases and asthma.

In macrobiotics, these are all symptoms of chronic imbalances in diet and lifestyle, which may lead to more serious illnesses. They are not viewed or treated as diseases or illnesses in and of themselves. All of these are a cumulative result of our dietary, activity and lifestyle practices. In fact, these symptoms are on the rise today as a result of poor diet and lack of contact with nature and physical activity.

Among the main contributors to blood-related disorders are:

1. Fast food, processed meat (including bacon), all dairy products, pizza, baked goods, refined foods, sugary foods, iced drinks, soft drinks.
2. These foods lead to excessive production of mucus and/or constriction of the bronchi, which makes it difficult to breathe out.
3. Lack of outdoor activity and insufficient contact with nature, especially from a young age.

Natural Ways of Elimination

Many degenerative illnesses are caused by the body's inability to eliminate or naturally discharge excess or toxins. The body has a natural, four-stage process of elimination.

1. Kidneys and Intestines
    Through daily urination and bowel movement, this is the
    healthiest way of cleansing the body.

2. Lungs
    When the body cannot eliminate toxins efficiently or
    thoroughly through the kidneys or intestines, it breaks
    down acidity to water and carbon dioxide, which are
    eliminated through the lungs along with excess mucus.

3. Skin
    The skin (in essence the third kidney) becomes involved
    if what needs eliminating can not get out otherwise.

4. Liver
    The liver tries to further neutralize acidity and detoxify.

What Is Asthma?

Asthma, from the macrobiotic viewpoint is a kidney
issue. It is associated with trouble in eliminating liquids
effectively or efficiently due to weak or stagnated kidneys.
The condition of the kidneys is related to diet and lifestyle.

Internal or external liquids commonly set off asthma
attacks. This includes sugary things that break down into
water and carbon dioxide, and cold, damp, or humid weather.

Asthma and the Environment

The quality of our haemoglobin sets the stage for our response
to external conditions such as pollen, pollution and other factors
like humidity. The condition of our blood determines how we
deal with, or respond to, environmental factors. Two people with

two different blood conditions will respond differently to the same environment. A healthy, alkaline condition of the blood increases the haemoglobin's ability to bind with and transport oxygen throughout the body, as well as to repel pollutants. As dietary and lifestyle habits worsen, these problems appear earlier during an individual's life cycle, even in young babies.

Macrobiotic Remedies to Relieve Asthma Symptoms

The best and long-term remedy is to ensure a healthy diet and lifestyle. In addition to this, try some of these macrobiotic remedies before resorting to steroidal bronchodilators.

1. Eat an umeboshi plum to neutralize acidity.
2. Kuzu with barley malt is a natural bronchodilator.
3. Black soybean tea is traditional oriental tea that opens and relaxes the bronchi.
4. Strong black coffee

Other Practices

Vigorous walks, especially in the morning, are very beneficial. The early morning sun helps to eliminate excess fluids in the body.

Body rubs aid circulation and make the process of elimination more efficient. Also, wear pure cotton to help the body breathe better.

Conclusion

The idea that asthma is caused solely because of genetics and the environment is disempowering to an individual. Asthma and allergies are symptoms of an overall imbalance that can be corrected through dietary and lifestyle change. Health allows us to be adaptable to various conditions and circumstances. Asthma is an early warning sign that our adaptability has been compromised. It is best to try and be more sensitive, listen to our body and respond with appropriate changes. There are countless individuals who have applied these principles and completely reversed asthma.

27

Asthma: Through the Looking Glass

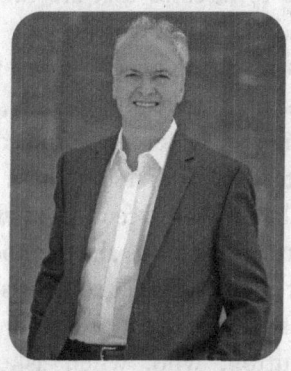

Tom Monte has written and co-authored more than thirty-five books on health, healing and personal transformation, including *Unexpected Recoveries: Seven Steps to Healing Body, Mind, and Soul When Serious Illness Strikes*. Find out more about Monte, his books and workshops by visiting his website, tommonte.com.

There is an old Sufi story about a man who loses his keys inside his house and decides to look for them under a street

lamp. When a neighbour passes by and asks his friend what
he is looking for, the man replies that he has lost his keys.

'Where did you lose them?'

'I lost them in the house.'

'Then why are you looking for them here on this corner?'

'Because the light is better out here.'

This humorous story tells us a lot about stubborn thinking,
which leads inevitably to failure.

A similar problem exists in medical science today.
Scientists and pharmaceutical companies are searching for
chemical solutions to diseases that are caused by poor diet,
lack of exercise and emotional distress.

Examples of this phenomenon are everywhere, but they
include epidemics of overweight, obesity, type-2 diabetes,
metabolic syndromes and several forms of cancer, just to
name a few. Instead of addressing these illnesses at their
cause, the medical and pharmaceutical establishments search
for chemical treatments—drugs that temporarily ameliorate
the symptoms but allow the cause to flourish.

This reminds me of a quote from American bank
robber Willie Sutton, who, when asked by a reporter
why he robbed banks, replied, 'Because that's where the
money is.'

As any pharmaceutical representative will tell you, the
money is in treatment, especially in treatments that do not
cure but keep people coming back for more. There's no
money in preventing a disease (that only reduces the market),
and there isn't much in curing it either. This explains why
very few illnesses are being cured by medical science today,
and why that trend will only continue.

Unfortunately, the approach to healthcare that's based
exclusively on short-term profit motive is leading us all to

disaster. If the current population of sick people doesn't shrink, and more people are added to the healthcare system, the system will be overrun with patients. That is exactly what is about to happen in the next thirty years, as hundreds of millions of obese, cancer-stricken, heart-diseased, Alzheimer-ridden diabetics overwhelm hospitals, medical offices, nursing homes and extended care facilities. Symptomatic medicine is about to meet its Waterloo.

These well-known epidemics challenge the limitations of medical thinking. But one disorder that presents medicine with an even more perplexing set of mysteries is asthma.

We cannot even begin to understand asthma, much less heal it, if we adhere to medical science's small definition of human life, which insists that basic biochemistry is all that matters when it comes to medicine and healthcare.

Asthma exists outside of these boundaries. It is rooted in the messy interplay between human psychology, emotions, biology and inherited constitutional strengths and weaknesses. In other words, it clearly involves all aspects of our humanity, which is why there's so little understanding about the disease.

Clues to a more accurate understanding of asthma, and a more effective set of treatments, do exist in medical literature. The problem is that these studies are largely ignored because they lead us into realms that reductionist scientists and doctors do not want to enter.

Asthma is the consequence, indeed the side effect, for how we cope with negative emotions, internal conflicts and beliefs about ourselves. When we find a cure for asthma, we'll have found the cure for modern life.

Like many other answers, that cure is out there, awaiting discovery. The question is: Are we willing to find it?

Asthma: Immune Reactions Block Oxygen

Asthma is a chronic condition that limits the afflicted person's ability to breathe. Periodic attacks of asthma can be very severe and even fatal. The incidence of asthma is rising throughout the world, but especially in First World nations.

Currently, there are approximately 300 million people worldwide who suffer from asthma. This number is expected to skyrocket over the next few decades. The disorder is especially widespread in the US, Great Britain, western Europe and Australia. The number of Americans afflicted with asthma (now 24 million) has doubled since the 1980s. In Great Britain, 10 per cent of children and 8 per cent of adults have asthma. On the other hand, it is virtually unheard of in many African nations.

The underlying condition that triggers asthma is inflammation. In other words, it is an immune reaction that causes the airways inside the lungs to become swollen and inflamed. As the tissues within these tubes swell, the passages become smaller and reduce air flow to the lungs.

Most people who suffer from asthma usually contract the condition in childhood, but the illness can arise at any age and is common among adults. On the other hand, many children who contract asthma discover that the illness passes when they reach adulthood, or becomes less severe.

Symptoms and Medical Treatment

The symptoms of asthma, which vary in severity and type, include difficulty in breathing, wheezing, sweating, rapid heart rate, great emotional distress, fear and anxiety. During an attack, the skin becomes pale and the lips may turn blue. For many, sleep is disturbed, shallow, or shortened.

Like all chronic conditions, asthma attacks rise suddenly, become acute and then recede. They can be triggered by an array of possible catalysts, including mold, animal dander, house dust, dust mites, cigarette smoke, air pollution, cockroach droppings and certain foods such as milk and milk products, eggs, peanuts, tree nuts, soy, wheat, fish and shellfish.

Asthma is an autoimmune disease where the person's own defense system turns against the body. Most treatments are designed to suppress the immune system, which in turn reduces the inflammation in the bronchioles. Among the drugs commonly used are albuterol (administered through an inhaler), corticosteroids and pharmaceutical drugs that can be taken intravenously (such as aminophyline).

Medical doctors state that there is no cure for asthma and that there are no methods for prevention. Treatment is focused primarily on asthma attacks, which is extremely important, given that people can die because of it. On the other hand, little effort is made to prevent it, perhaps because there is so little understanding of the illness. Maybe that is why the numbers keep going up worldwide.

If we open up our view of ourselves and find a way to join modern science with ancient wisdom, we can gain insights into the causes and cures of asthma. We can also see more deeply into our own humanness.

Asthma Is an Emotionally-Based Disorder

Somehow, we in the West decided that emotions are irrelevant to healthcare. Common sense tells us otherwise, but we've been blinded to that old-fashioned faculty. This explains why so much research that shows that asthma is directly linked to anger, depression and fear has been dismissed by clinicians and researchers alike.

In any event, the case for linking the onset of asthma and asthma attacks with our emotional life is a strong one. For example, in a study published in the medical journal *Thorax* (October 2006, 61 [10:863-8]), researchers from the Harvard School of Public Health examined the effects of anger and hostility on the lung function of 670 men. The study was a prospective experiment, meaning the researchers measured the degree of anger and hostility in the men first and then determined the effects these emotions had on their lungs. Not surprisingly, the researchers found that anger and hostility significantly reduced overall lung function, narrowing airways and contributing to overall decline.

'This overall association between higher hostility and reduced lung function remained significant after adjusting for smoking and education,' the researchers found. 'Higher hostility was associated with a more rapid decline in lung function and this effect was unchanged and remained significant . . .' Not only did anger and hostility reduce the ability of the men to breathe, but these emotions also contributed to the decline of the lungs over time.

In a similar study, German scientists from the University of Hamburg studied the effects of emotions on asthmatics and non-asthmatics. The researchers showed two groups— one composed of people with asthma and another composed of non-asthmatics. They showed both groups photographs depicting emotionally charged imagery. Each photograph was meant to evoke a different emotional state. After showing them the photographs, the scientists measured the effects of these emotional states on the air passages in the lungs. They were also able to measure the effects of one's mood on breathing in both groups. The photographs that evoked negative emotions such as anger, fear and hostility, affected lung function in both groups, but more severely in the asthmatic patients.

'Unpleasant mood is associated with decreased respiratory function in asthmatic patients in everyday life and in laboratory assessments,' the scientists concluded. But the fact that these images affected both groups is worth noting. It's possible— even likely—that most of us experience some degree of lung dysfunction after experiencing or witnessing an unpleasant event. But some of our lungs are more sensitive to trauma and thus more vulnerable to an asthmatic reaction.

Stanford University researchers examined the effects of different moods stimulated by watching films in the laboratory. The results showed that not only did negative mood and emotional states significantly reduce lung function, but positive emotions also lowered lung function in the asthmatics, though not as much as the negative emotions. The Stanford researchers also found that the asthmatics were particularly susceptible to depression.

The researchers, who published their study in *Psychosomatic Medicine* (November–December 2000, 62 [6:808–15]), concluded that 'pulmonary function of asthmatic patients is negatively affected by strong mood states in daily life. Airway effects of negative emotion . . . particularly depression, can predict changes in pulmonary function in response to negative mood . . .'

The reference to depression is important because other researchers have found that many asthmatics are particularly susceptible to depression. Mexican researchers studied 85 children with asthma and found that '100 percent of the evaluated asthmatic children and adolescents showed [mood states] related to depression'.

After a review of medical literature, scientists from Robert Wood Johnson Medical School in New Jersey reported in a 1993 issue of *Journal of Asthma* that 'asthmatics tend to report and display a high level of negative emotion, and asthma exacerbations [i.e., asthma attacks] have been linked temporarily to periods of heightened emotionality.'

In fact, medical literature is bursting with studies showing that heightened negative emotions—anger, fear and depression—are among the most common characteristics shared by people with asthma. Moreover, asthma attacks arise when these underlying emotional states flare and cause dramatic changes in lung function, which in turn cause the narrowing of the bronchioles and severely affect breathing.

Children Feel Greatly but Cannot Speak their Truth

One of the important lessons every healer learns early in his or her training is that emotions are, in fact, bundles of energy that cause dramatic change in biochemistry, and organ and muscle function. Also, emotions have tremendous power to cause physical contractions or relaxation.

For example, take shock and fear. If a child is sitting on the floor with a crayon, colouring a picture, and an adult suddenly screams at him or her in anger, the child will go into a state of shock that will trigger an array of changes in the body. The most obvious symptom will be an instantaneous contraction of virtually every muscle. An array of other biochemical changes will also occur, including the release of stress hormones, such as cortisol, which is a primary cause of inflammation.

The truth is that many children are shocked on a regular basis by traumatic events or sudden emotional outbursts from parents, teachers and siblings. Many children are verbally, physically, and/or sexually abused as well. These are the more obvious sources of trauma. But there are subtle forms of emotional injury that tend to be overlooked such as regular arguments between parents, a depressed parent, parents who are struggling with illness, fear of job loss, or some other tragedy that cannot be avoided.

In fact, most families are forced to deal with challenges and tragedies over which they have no control. Parents do their best to protect their children from the difficulties adults face, but very few of us have effective coping mechanisms. We do our best, but our children feel every bit of our pain. And they suffer with us.

Children are so attuned to the emotional lives of their parents that they cannot help but experience, in very intimate ways, the internal conflicts and turmoil that their parents experience. This means that not only must children cope with their own emotional distress, but they must also deal with the weight of their family's turmoil. Consequently, as stress hormones rise, the immune system goes into action. Inflammation rises throughout the system, including in the lungs.

The terrible conundrum that children face is that they cannot speak the truth, tell their stories, and express their pain. Yes, they lack the vocabulary, but more importantly, they lack the awareness of what is happening. Meanwhile, adults too do not encourage their children to speak the truth or purge their frustration, anger and fear in a healthy way.

In fact, in most cases, adults ask children to cope with their emotional pain by 'being good', or 'learning to behave', which is our code for asking them to make fewer demands of us. Children realize this and very often adopt a pattern of silence, especially when it comes to their own needs and experiences.

Their stories their challenges at school and home, with friends, or in their neighbourhoods remain buried inside of them, causing patterns of distress that become deeply imbedded. They linger and fester, ready to implode or explode, depending on the nature of the child.

When emotions—especially shock, fear and anger—go unexpressed and unhealed, they can have long-term effects on stress hormones, inflammation, muscle contraction and altered states of organ function. Our bodies are literally reshaped by the emotional events and traumas of our youth.

It's possible that the science of post-traumatic stress, which is still in its infancy, will one day help us understand the degrees of trauma each of us carry. What we do know is that trauma creates a kind of emotional and biological programming which is set in motion every time we experience some degree of stress. For many of us, that programming triggers the same biochemical and emotional cascade, no matter how severe the stressor may be. This is why so many of us overreact to relatively minor events. Even small triggers can set off our underlying programming and thus set the cascade in motion.

For a sensitive child—whose lungs are particularly vulnerable—these patterns of stress, emotion (especially anger) and silence change the way the lungs function. This may well be the basis for asthma. In fact, this is also true for adults who struggle with asthma.

The two emotions that have the greatest power to trigger this traumatic programming are anger and fear. This is especially true of a certain form of anger, which I refer to as powerless anger.

Powerless Anger Is at the Root of Asthma

One of the most difficult emotions for any family to deal with is anger. In many families, only one member is allowed to be angry. Usually, that person is the father. He is, after all, coping with the world and earning a living—that's the rationale used to justify the rage. In many families, however, it's the mother who is angry and the father who is passive.

Anger can exist without necessarily exploding into verbal or physical violence. Lots of angry people merely seethe or become withdrawn, manipulative, passive–aggressive, or withhold their love. Anger can take on many forms. The more powerless an angry person feels the more indirect, manipulative and unjust he becomes. People with powerless anger invariably take out their rage on innocent people, usually on dependents.

When one family member is angry and everyone else is silent, it means that all the other members are forced to repress their anger and their power and personal experiences. They swallow their rage, bury their truth and make excuses for one or both parents. Meanwhile, they feel powerless to change the one person who is allowed to be angry. They are also afraid of expressing their own anger for fear that they will be punished or attacked or will lose all hope of gaining their parents' love.

Anger within the family is always accompanied by fear. We are angry at one or both parents, afraid of his or her wrath and afraid that we will never receive his or her love. Hence, children repress their anger to get along, keep their hopes alive and survive.

This anger only gets worse in adulthood. That our world is becoming angrier is proof of this statement. Too many adults are feeling powerless to affect positive change in their lives. Gun sales have risen and not because people feel good about themselves, or their neighbours. We have lost faith in the power of our words and the dignity of our bearing. And virtually everyone—children and adults alike—deal with anger in the same way: with food.

Food is among the primary means of dampening emotional turmoil. The food that is the cause of asthma are the foods that children use most often as anaesthetics for their emotional pain—sugar, soft drinks, processed foods and dairy products such as ice cream, cheese, butter and yogurt.

Food Is a Primary Source of Inflammation

All the foods we use to cope with stress, fear, anger, frustration and depression are highly inflammatory. Processed foods, including sugar, white flour products and soft drinks all cause rapid elevations in blood glucose and insulin, which in turn increase weight and trigger the release of highly inflammatory compounds, including tumour necrosis factor (TNC) and interleukin-6 (Il-6).

Milk products contain insulin-like growth factor (IGF-1), which is highly inflammatory. Milk proteins and purines also trigger immune reactions and lead to inflammation, especially in milk-sensitive children and adults. Milk proteins also elevate homocysteine, which acts on soft tissues—including those in the lungs—like battery acid. The injury caused by homocysteine triggers an immune reaction in the sensitive tissues, which in turn causes inflammation.

The saturated fat in animal products drives up blood cholesterol levels, which triggers an immune reaction in all the places where cholesterol plaques collect, especially in the arteries around the heart and in the lungs.

The combination of highly toxic emotions—especially anger, fear and depression—with highly toxic foods—especially processed foods and dairy products—is the real cause of asthma.

Ancient Wisdom, Modern Needs

Our ancestral healers understood the union of psychological states, emotions, food and physical constitution in ways that modern minds have great difficulty appreciating. Perhaps the most advanced system for articulating this union of body, mind and spirit was the Chinese system of the Five Transformations.

The Five Transformations articulated how organs rely upon each other in order to function optimally. No organ functions exclusively. Rather, it depends on other organs for support.

In the case of asthma, the lungs are dependent upon the spleen, kidneys and liver. When it comes to treating asthma, these organs are key. This becomes clear when we understand that the Chinese maintained that each organ holds and is responsible for regulating a specific emotional state. A brief summary of that system follows:

1. The lungs hold and regulate sadness and grief. Conversely, the lungs are injured by excessive sadness and grief.
2. The kidneys and bladder regulate fear, courage and innate will power. They are affected by excessive fear.
3. The liver is associated with anger, frustration, emotional balance and the expression of our will and deep feelings. The more anger there is in one's life, the greater the insult and injury to the liver.

4. The heart is linked to joy. When the heart is imbalanced, the emotional state becomes chaotic and we experience hysteria. The more chaos there is in one's life, the greater the injury to the heart.
5. The spleen, stomach and pancreas hold and regulate compassion and empathy. These organs also strengthen our sense of self and our boundaries. When the spleen and stomach become weak, we over-identify with the feelings of others, which can result in a loss of one's sense of self and a loss of one's connection with his or her truth. Over-identification with other people injures the spleen, stomach and pancreas.

As an organ weakens, the negative emotional state becomes more pronounced. These emotions are heightened in the case of an asthmatic, which indicates that all associated organs are in a weakened state. They must all be treated in order to heal asthma.

Meanwhile, the excessive and imbalanced emotions within the body must also be released and healed. In other words, the trauma-programming, with its emotional and biological cascade, must be transformed in order to heal asthma.

What to Do?

Pharmaceutical drugs, including inhalers and other forms of medication, will go on being necessary as long as the person with asthma goes on reacting to negative emotions and stressful events with the same emotional and biochemical cascade.

In order to transform that programming, we must learn to react to stressful events and negative emotions in a different manner. In effect, we must break the old habit of swallowing our emotions and turning anger in on ourselves. At the same time, we must stop using the same poisonous foods to cope with stress and negative emotions.

Four steps must be followed if we are to transform the underlying, trauma-based programming. These are:

1. We must undergo regular healing touch or acupuncture in order to release the effects of emotional stress that are still being carried in our organs and tissues, especially in the lungs, kidneys and liver. The tension and trauma held in these organs are still triggering that inflammatory cascade that is at the root of the asthma.

2. We must stop consuming refined white sugar and all dairy products, including milk, cheese, yogurt and ice cream. We must also sharply reduce processed foods, which cause both glucose and insulin spikes, both of which lead to higher levels of inflammation. These foods may act as temporary analgesics for emotional distress, but they in fact fuel the biochemical cascade that leads to inflammation and asthma. Replace sugar with cooked fruit and foods sweetened with rice syrup, barley malt, maple syrup and cooked apple juice. Eat sweet vegetables such as squash, carrots, onion and pumpkin.

3. We must practise speaking our truths and expressing our emotions in safe environments, such as writing them in a diary and speaking to therapists and healers. This must be done consistently and habitually. Rather than suppressing our emotions, they must be expressed outwardly. That outward expression must lead to new behaviours in which we feel a growing sense of our power and control in life.

4. We must add foods to our diet that heal the lungs, kidneys, liver and spleen.

In order to heal the lungs, eat:

1. Leafy vegetables, especially collard greens, mustard greens, bok choy, Chinese cabbage and green cabbage.
2. White vegetables, especially daikon, onion, turnip and cauliflower.
3. Boiled brown rice. Eat brown rice once or twice a day for three or four days per week.
4. Small amounts (half a teaspoon) of fresh grated ginger, twice a week, in vegetable medleys and soups.
5. Mochi, or pounded sweet rice, in soups with green and leafy vegetables once or twice a week.

In order to heal the kidneys:

1. Substitute vegetable proteins for animal proteins during most meals.
2. Eat beans daily, especially aduki beans, black beans, navy and kidney beans. Eat tempeh and tofu as substitutes for beans, but make beans the priority.
3. Eat sea vegetables such as arame, wakame, and sushi nori daily. Sea vegetables, rich in minerals, alkalize the blood and support the kidneys.
4. Restrict animal foods to fish once or twice a week and one or two eggs, twice a month, until the asthma attacks are alleviated.
5. Eat root vegetables, especially burdock, carrots, parsnips, lotus root and rutabaga.

6. Eat buckwheat as groats and as pasta, such as soba noodles in tamari or shoyu broth.

7. Eat a small amount of pickles three to five times per week after dinner meal. Pickles alkalize the blood and provide digestive enzymes.

8. Eat miso soup four to six times per week. Miso soup should include wakame seaweed, along with small amounts of green and root vegetables.

9. Eat black sesame seeds as a condiment on cooked grains and vegetables.

10. Eat chestnuts in fall and winter, and watermelon in summer.

11. Use sea salt in cooking (usually a pinch is all that is needed).

12. Avoid all cold and iced drinks.

13. Avoid excess protein, especially from animal foods, especially red meat and dairy products.

14. Avoid table salt.

28

Yoga for Asthma

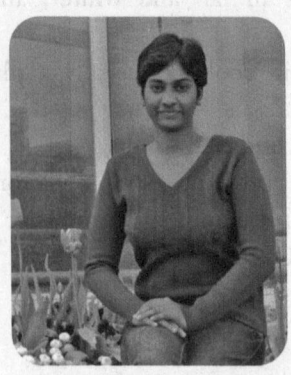

Dr Suma Bentur, B.A.M.S., D.Y.T., is an Ayurveda doctor and a certified yoga expert who has conducted several workshops in India and abroad. Dr Bentur distils her eighteen years of experience and knowledge to guide you on your health journey with lifestyle, diet, herbs and yoga practices that help you heal, prevent diseases and achieve optimal health. Her treatment protocols for individuals are customized and comprehensive.

Ayurveda and yoga view asthma as a multi-systemic disease that is caused due to a weak digestive system, creating *ama* or biotoxins that spread from the gastrointestinal tract to the lungs causing respiratory distress. Also, the respiratory system is greatly influenced by an individual's state of mind, metabolism and excretory functions.

Yoga as a therapy offers a corrective and curative approach, strengthening the digestive system, lungs and the bronchiole lining. Various researches have empirically proven that yogic practices bring about qualitative improvement by reducing the severity and duration of an asthma attack.

Yoga asanas help release muscular tension around the ribs and improve respiratory stamina—pranayama increases the breathing capacity and reduces the hypersensitivity of airways. Shat kriyas or cleansing techniques, performed under the strict supervision and guidance of a certified yoga teacher, help re-vitalize an asthamatic's power of digestion and relieves constipation.

Stress and anxiety can worsen an asthamatic's symptoms. Meditation and deep relaxation techniques can help improve the functioning of their airways and respiratory muscles.

The following asanas and pranayama practices with meditation are beneficial for those suffering from respiratory ailments.

Ardhakati Chakrasana	The pose brings balance to the entire body. It stretches the muscles between the ribs and the pelvis and opens the sides of the chest cavity. The bending action helps you breathe better.
Padahastasana	This posture tones the abdominal organs and stabilizes the apana vayu, thereby nourishing the excretory system, and enhancing the digestive system and metabolism. It also has a calming effect on the mind.

Ardha Chakrasana	It massages and stretches the colon and abdominal organs, thus improving digestion. It improves one's lung capacity and is beneficial for those with respiratory disorders.
Trikonasana	This pose activates the rib cage and stretches the intercostal muscles.
Vakrasana or Ardha Matsyendrasana	Vakrasana is a very effective pose to tone your abdomen and stretch your thighs. It can help cure and prevent constipation and indigestion.
Bhujangasana	This expands the chest and increases the lung capacity. It is ideal for people with asthma and respiratory congestion.
Pavan Muktasana	This asana helps eliminate excess gas in the stomach and works on the digestive system. The abdominal compression it creates relieves constipation and other issues caused by the imbalance of Vata dosha, which is the root cause of asthma.
Matsyasana	Matsyasna works on the muscles around the neck, chest and lumbar region. It relieves respiratory problems by encouraging proper breathing.
Shavasana	This pose is done mostly at the end of yoga practices. It influences deep relaxation that helps asthmatics deal with their symptoms associated with anxiety and stress.

Pranayama Practices

Practices like Nadi Shuddhi, Bhramari and chanting 'aum' have found a mention in numerous studies. The benefits they offer include:

1. Improving lung function.
2. Skeletal muscle strength.
3. Strength of expiratory as well as inspiratory muscles.

4. Reduces exercise-induced bronchoconstriction.
5. Reduced hypersensitivity of the airways, making asthmatics more resistant to allergens.

29

Healing Asthma

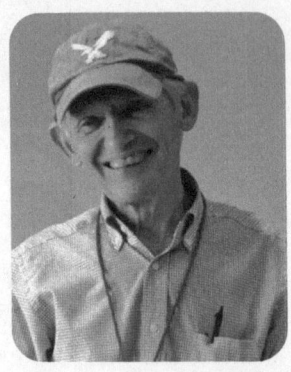

Alex Jack is an author, teacher and dietary counsellor. He is the president of Planetary Health and a sponsor of Amberwaves and the Macrobiotic Summer Conference. His books include *The Cancer-Prevention* Diet with Michio Kushi and *The One Peaceful World Cookbook* with Sachi Kato. He co-hosts the *Miso Happy Show*, an online variety programme with Bettina Zumdick. Alex lives in the Berkshires in Massachusetts.

Asthma is caused primarily by dairy food that blocks or impedes respiration. It is also associated with pollution and

318

other contaminants that can get into the lungs. People with asthma suffer from an airway inflammation and are sensitive to certain triggers. Some people experience an asthma attack during different seasons and because of certain environmental pollutants, allergens (dust, chemicals, and drugs), irritants or food additives. A cold or a bout of bronchitis may also trigger an asthma attack. Another trigger may be exercise or sports or anxiety.

Symptoms

Wheezing and coughing are common symptoms. The wheezing may begin suddenly and worsen at night, after exercise, or after being exposed to cold air. Also, one may experience a tightening of the chest or shortness of breath. Coughing up blood, a brief lapse in breathing and when exhaling takes much longer that inhaling are less common symptoms.

Treatments

Asthma attacks can be dangerous and need to be watched very closely. We can try to relieve them by applying ginger compresses to the chest, in the front as well as in the back. Compresses may need to be repeated, sometimes for up to one or several hours, before an attack fades away.

You could also try this specific drink: crush 20 grams of peach kernels and 12 grams of apricot kernels in a suribachi. Add some grated ginger and a little rice malt, and boil this together with water for 5–10 minutes. Drink and eat everything.

In the short term it may be that the intake of something yin will have an effect, such as hot water with rice honey, or kuzu with barley malt, or hot apple juice; some people notice relief after drinking strong coffee. This may relieve the attack and can safely be used at that time, but if this would be the only treatment in the long term, it would gradually worsen the condition and lead to sooner and more serious attacks.

To treat the cause of asthma, one should try to become more yang by using a standard macrobiotic diet together with a moderate intake of gomashio (home-made sesame salt) or umeboshi plums.

Bibliography

1. *The Complete Macrobiotic Diet: Seven Steps to Feel Fabulous, Look Vibrant, and Think Clearly*, Denny Waxman and Susan Waxman.
2. *Macrobiotics for Dummies*, Verne Varona.
3. *Unexpected Recoveries, Seven Steps to Healing Body, Mind, and Soul When Serious Illness Strikes*, Tom Monte.
4. *The Cancer Prevention Diet*, Alex Jack and Michio Kushi.
5. *Yin Yang Primer*, Edward Esko.
6. *Contemporary Macrobiotics*, Edward Esko.
7. *Rice Field Essays*, Edward Esko.
8. *Dandelion Essays*, Edward Esko.
9. *Ki: The Energy of Life*, Edward Esko.
10. *Opening Your Third Eye*, Edward Esko.
11. *Authentic Foods: Health Benefits of Whole Foods, Facts, Recipes and More*, Bettina Zumdick.
12. *The One Peaceful World Cookbook*, Sachi Kato and Alex Jack.
13. *Nature's Cancer-Fighting Foods*, Verne Varona.
14. *Delicious Desserts for all Occasions*, Bettina Zumdick.
15. *The Hip Chick's Guide to Macrobiotics*, Jessica Porter.

16. *Macrobiotics for All Seasons*, Marlene Watson-Tara.
17. *Yummy Yummy in my Tummy*, Melanie Waxman.
18. *The Self Healing Cookbook*, Kristina Turner.
19. *Modern-Day Macrobiotics*, Simon G. Brown.
20. *Eat Me Now*, Melanie Brown Waxman.
21. *Beautiful Children: The Parent's Essential Guide to Raising Strong, Balanced, Healthy Children*, Tarika Ahuja.

Resources

Since I live in Delhi–NCR, here are a few stores/farms I am familiar with:

1) For urban farming and developing, or home kitchen gardens, visit: http://www.edibleroutes.com.
2) I Say Organic, https://www.isayorganic.com/.
3) The Roots, Organic Lifestyle Store, https://www.organicstoretheroots.in/.
4) Live Organic, https://www.liveorganic.co.in/.
5) The Altitude Store, http://www.thealtitudestore.com/.
6) Navdanya, http://www.navdanya.org/site/.

For more organic stores across India, you can look up the eSvasa yellow organic pages.

Recommendations:

1) Keep organic apple juice by 24 Letter Mantra (http://www.24mantra.com/) handy in your house. After consulting your doctor, have hot apple juice for immediate relief from an asthma attack.

2) Try Wakaba products for therapeutic-grade Japanese ingredients used in some recipes listed in Chapter 24. They carry high-quality unadulterated Japanese foods (without MSG and other harmful chemicals).

Suggestions if You Want to Study Macrobiotics:

1) For an excellent online professional one-year certified programme (MYH–Master Your Health) and other short-term programmes, look up Strengthening Health Institute (SHI) on https://shimacrobiotics.org/.
2) For the yearly macrobiotic summer conference, usually held in west Massachusetts, and winter online programmes, visit https://www.macrobioticsummerconference.com/.
3) For short-term and long-term programmes in natural healing, visit https://tommonte.com/.
4) For short workshops and online medicinal cooking programmes, visit http://www.culinarymedicineschool.com/.

Recommendations for Online One-to-One Wellness and Health Consultants:

1) Denny Waxman, https://dennywaxman.com/.
2) Tom Monte, https://tommonte.com/.
3) Verne Varona, https://www.vernevarona.com/.
4) Bettina Zumdick, https://www.culinarymedicineschool.com/.
5) Edward Esko, https://www.internationalmacrobioticinstitute.com/.

Acknowledgements

I would like to thank my parents, my brother, my sister-in-law, my friends, supportive neighbours and extended family, especially my thoughtful and supportive cousins. A special thanks to my mother for supporting me throughout the processes of writing this book. I would also like to acknowledge my father for supporting me with his time, constructive feedback and financial aid for many months so I could concentrate effectively on this project. Many thanks to my nephews Owen, Jai and Sannat, and nieces Vivani, Ruksaana, Jhanvi, Sanam, Naiya and Samya. Seeing the new generation in my family inspires me to present information in a way that is easy and structured for them to use and something they hopefully share with their family and friends someday.

A heartfelt thanks to warm-hearted guides, inspiring friends and teachers—Kabir and Meena Chawla, Denny and Susan Waxman, Edward Esko, Bettina Zumdick, Tom and Toby Monte, Alex Jack, Verne Varona, David Kerr, Shruti Poddar, Dr Jairam Nair, Sajan Narain, late Mona Shwartz and many other members of the macrobiotic and yoga community that I am blessed to be part of. Many thanks are also due to

Denny Waxman, Tom Monte, Dr Suma Bentur and Alex
Jack for contributing article to my book. Their participation
in my book inspires me to spread their valuable wisdom and
message to everyone.

Gratitude to all those who have thoughtfully and
generously sent me their recipes for the section on international
recipes: Bettina Zumdick, Susan Waxman, Susan Ragsdale,
Anna Aeschlimann, Susan Beram, Sylvia Ruth Gray, Alex
Garberg, Masumi Goldman, Amber Maisano, Simone
Parris, Kezia Snyder and Carol Wasserman. Thank you to
my friends Swati Newatia, Tanveer Kaur, Atul Johri, Vivek
Ghai and Ma Prem Bhakti for their support and feedback.

I would also like to thank I Say Organic for their altruistic
work and the vegetables they gifted for the photoshoot of this
book. Many thanks are due to Roots Organic for their support
in helping me spread my message, and for their consistently
good work.

I would also like to extend a very special thank you to
Gaurav Shrinagesh, Gurveen Chadha and the entire team at
Penguin Random House India for understanding and trusting
my message and intention to support people suffering from
asthma and other lung-related diseases. Last, but not the least,
thank you to all those who read this book and apply the health
principles and practical steps it offers, and set an example of
healing with natural foods and lifestyle for everyone around.

Scan QR code to access the
Penguin Random House India website